PULP CAVITIES OF THE PERMANENT TEETH

An Anatomical Guide to Manipulative Endodontics

RUSSELL C. WHEELER, D.D.S., F.A.C.D.

Washington University School of Dentistry
    Instructor, Crown and Bridge Prosthesis, 1924–1927
    Instructor, Dental Anatomy and Prosthetic Art, 1927–1935
    Assistant Professor, Oral Anatomy, 1936
Washington University School of Dentistry
    Associate Professor of Anatomy, 1945–1951
    Research Professor, Dental Anatomy and Physiology, 1971–1974
St. Louis University School of Dentistry
    Associate Professor of Dental Anatomy, Human and Comparative,
    Chairman of Department, 1937–1944
Washington University School of Dentistry
    Associate Professor of Anatomy, 1945–1951
    Research Professor, Dental Anatomy and Physiology, 1971–
Washington University School of Dentistry
    Visiting Lecturer and Research Professor in Dental
    Anatomy and Physiology, 1974–

1976

W. B. SAUNDERS COMPANY • Philadelphia • London • Toronto

W. B. Saunders Company: West Washington Square
                          Philadelphia, Pa. 19105

                          12 Dyott Street
                          London, WC1A 1DB

                          833 Oxford Street
                          Toronto, Ontario M8Z 5T9, Canada

Library of Congress Cataloging in Publication Data
Wheeler, Russell Charles.
Pulp cavities of the permanent teeth.
Includes index.
1. Endodontics.   2. Dental pulp cavity.   I. Title. [DNLM: 1. Dental pulp cavity — Anatomy and histology — Atlases.   2. Root canal therapy — Atlases. WU17 W564p]
RK351.W48   617.6'34   74-25483
ISBN 0-7216-9280-X

Pulp Cavities of the Permanent Teeth: ISBN 0-7216-9280-X
An Anatomical Guide to Manipulative Endodontics

Last digit is the print number: 9   8   7   6   5   4   3   2   1

Preface

As mentioned in Chapter 1, which is designed as an introduction to this book, *Pulp Cavities of the Permanent Teeth* provides much valuable information previously unstudied in the endodontic literature. Studies in tooth morphology which feature cross sections of the teeth have been neglected. At present, the pulp cavity anatomy is poorly illustrated, even in excellent books on endodontics. The subject treated here in atlas form imparts information mainly by means of illustrations. Each chapter will have an introductory text, rather condensed, dealing with the physical approach to treatment. Originally, of course, all endodontic treatment by general practitioners in dentistry, was "physical." How "clean" and "sterile" one could get a given pulp cavity before filling to the "very end" of the root indicated the excellence of results. Today, of course, it is taken for granted that the "physical approach" is not sufficient. However, the anatomical truisms are recognized as important, because unless future research dictates otherwise, the more perfect the ultimate filling of root spaces is, the more perfect the treatment expectations are likely to be. This preface will include some of the information presented in Chapter 1:

The specialty of endodontics (which can be appreciated by general practitioners in dentistry) demands that more attention be paid to the macroscopic approach to diagnosis and prognosis when planning endodontic treatment. The successful manipulation of instruments clinically will require instinctive dexterity based on a thorough knowledge of probable anatomical features. Education in dental anatomy with special emphasis on root form is of primary importance.

The plan of this atlas is to review pulp cavity morphology and to show its relevance in clinical dentistry. Chapters describe the anatomy of and endodontic approach to specific individual permanent teeth, singly or in pairs. The sequence of their consideration is governed by the indicators of practical experience; those presented first are the teeth most likely to require treatment earlier in life.

Only part of this information will be included in the written text. Actually, the introductory text to each chapter will give only a short résumé of the anatomical characteristics of the tooth or teeth in question. It will mention possibilities of normalcy or abnormality and whether or not unusual problems in endodontic treatment are to be expected. The condensed text will be followed by enlarged photos (in most instances); these graphic illustrations, arranged in logical sequence and accompanied by descriptive legends, will complete the planned instruction in the subject covered by the chapter.

Those involved with the endodontic approach in treatment will be concerned primarily with root formations. Strange as it may seem, a detailed study of root forms is often neglected in the dental school curriculum. Therefore, early in each chapter root forms will be featured. The facial and mesial aspects of uncut tooth specimens will be provided. These enlarged photos will show a typical pulp cavity form painted on the respective tooth surfaces. This learning approach helps the operator to form a mental picture of the probable pulp cavity form to be encountered after the occlusal approach is made to the pulp chamber in the tooth to be treated (Fig. 2–10).

Many of the illustrations included in each chapter may not be referred to in the introductory text. They will follow in sequence in a manner that will be of reader interest; each figure is also accompanied by a descriptive legend, some quite extensive. Each one may stand alone as a graphic illustration of its pulp cavity involvement in endodontics.

RUSSELL C. WHEELER

Contents

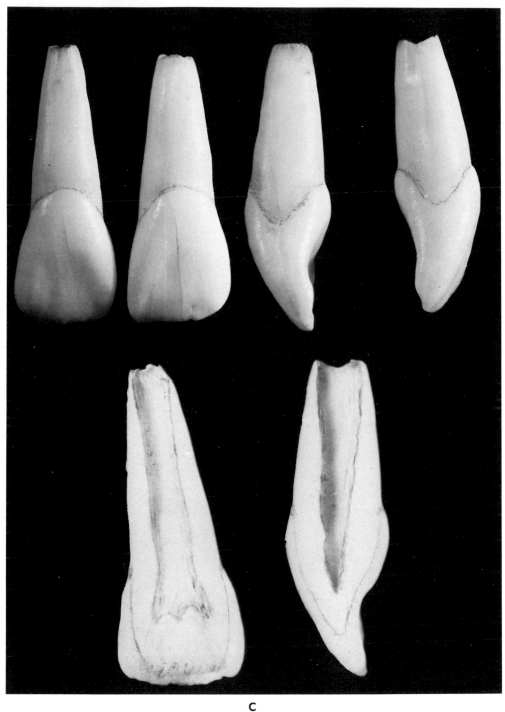

Figure 1–1 Maxillary central incisors. This case afforded an unusual opportunity to study separate cross sections of the "same tooth"; further explanation will be forthcoming in Chapter 1.

A, Labial aspect of matched central incisors.

B, Mesial and distal aspects of the incisors.

C, The central incisors after sectioning: left, mesiodistal cross section; right, labiolingual cross section. Note the space for pulp horns in the mesiodistal section.

Introduction

Endodontics has been favored in the past with detailed studies covering microbiology, pharmacology, and related subjects, including oral and dental anatomy. In the literature, however, the study of the morphology of permanent teeth viewed in cross section has been limited.

The specialty of endodontics demands that more attention be paid to the macroscopic approach to diagnosis and prognosis when planning such treatment. The successful manipulation of instruments clinically requires instinctive dexterity based on a thorough knowledge of probable anatomical features. Education in dental anatomy with special emphasis on root form is of primary importance.

The dental pulp is centered in the dentin body of the tooth; the anatomical outline form of the pulp cavity will be a reflection of the outer form of the dentin body, whether it be viewed faciolingually or mesiodistally in cross section. The pulp cavity measurements will be smaller, of course, but will have similar relative dimensions (Fig. 1–2). Therefore, the first rule for establishing a mental image of the pulp tissue and pulp cavity form is to be able to recall the overall form of the tooth in question from any angle.

Those interested in dental restoration will be concerned mainly with crown form, whereas those involved with the endodontic approach in treatment will have root formations uppermost in mind. Strange as it may seem, a detailed study of root forms is often neglected in the dental school curriculum. This book will place special emphasis on root forms and their significance in establishing pulp cavity design.

Two fields in dentistry that require particular attention to pulp cavity anatomy are clinical operative dentistry and endodontics. Cavity preparation and the preparation of crown portions in crown or fixed appliance techniques will presuppose a thorough knowledge of pulp chamber size and shape. A pulp cavity may be large, as in young individuals, or it may be shrunken and constricted by excessive formation of secondary dentin; there may be calcification within the pulp tissue itself (Fig. 3–1). The operator should make a thorough diagnosis of the situation before beginning any treatment procedure.

Because the primary purpose of this book is to present studies in macroscopic anatomy, there will be no attempt to compete with excellent works covering the subjects of oral histology and embryology, which treat thoroughly the development and function of pulp tissue. These topics will be mentioned only as they affect the anatomy of the pulp cavities with respect to the macroscopic approach taken here.

In the discussion of any scientific subject, appeal must be directed to the novice as well as to the specialist. Therefore, this introductory chapter is somewhat simplified, repeating information that to more learned and sophisticated readers may seem elementary and obvious. The author's objective is to attract the attention of anyone interested in pulp cavity design, regardless of the reader's category in dentistry.

THE PULP CAVITIES OF THE PERMANENT TEETH

The dental pulp is the soft tissue component of the tooth. It is a connective tissue originating from the mesenchyme of the dental papilla, and it performs multiple functions throughout life. It is the formative organ of the dentin as well as the source of nutrition and maintenance of the dentin. One of the pulp's most important functions is sensory and defensive; if the tooth is exposed to any irritation which the pulp detects, it will produce a very definite defense reaction which could serve as a warning of impending problems.

For study of the anatomy of pulp cavities in teeth, longitudinal sections of each tooth, both faciolingually and mesiodistally, should be made. In addition, transverse sections should be prepared with cuts through the crowns or roots at various levels. As mentioned previously, these dissections expose a central cavity with an outline corresponding in general to that of the dentin body. *This space is called the pulp cavity,* and in life it contains the dental pulp (Fig. 1–3). That portion of the pulp cavity found mainly within the coronal portion of the tooth is the pulp chamber, while the remainder, found within the root, is called the pulp canal. The constricted opening of the pulp canal at the root end is the apical foramen. It is possible for any tooth root to have more than one foramen; in such cases, the canals have two or more branches that make their exits at or near the apical end of the root. These may be called multiple foramina or supplementary canals (Figs. 1–4 and 1–9, *A*).

The pulp chamber is centered in the crown and is always a single cavity. The pulp canals of roots are continuous with this cavity. Many roots are found with more than one canal. The mesial root of the mandibular first molar, for instance, may contain two pulp canals; these two canals, however, may end in a common foramen (Fig. 3–6, *A*, 1, 2).

To repeat, the shape of the pulp chamber varies with the shape of the crown. Also, when the roots are much wider in one direction than in another, the pulp canal forms will vary accordingly. Since the crowns of the teeth are wider in all measurements than the root forms, and the roots taper from the root trunk to the apices, the pulp cavities taper from their largest measurement within the crown to a final constriction at the apical foramen. Sometimes the canals are so constricted as they approach the apical terminal that it is very difficult to avoid obliterating them while making cross sections of specimens (Fig. 7–23).

The size of the pulp cavity will be influenced by the age of the tooth, its functional activity, and its history. The dental pulp decreases in size gradually as the tooth ages. Therefore, the youngest teeth are provided with the largest, most open pulp cavities (Figs. 1–1 and 3–1, *A*).

Figure 1–1 shows photographs of twin permanent maxillary central incisors, in a female aged 6½ years, that were lost in an unfortunate accident. *A* and *B* in the illustration show the matched incisors before they were sectioned. Since they seemed to be identical in form, one could be sectioned mesiodistally and the other labiolingually, thereby presenting for study separate cross sections of the "same tooth."

In Figure 1–1, *C* the sectioned specimens are shown. The mesiodistal cross section on the left shows a wide, rather formless pulp cavity overall but having three distinct pulp horn formations. In contrast, the labiolingual cross section on the right shows the variation in pulp cavity design from this aspect. Here the cavity tapers rapidly toward the crown and comes to a point in the center of the crown. The root ends are, of course, incomplete, but the roots are nearer their final length than is usually the case for central incisors in one so young. It is true, however, that girls are in advance of boys in dental development schedules.

Throughout its life the dental pulp retains the ability to deposit what is called secondary dentin, ostensibly for its protection; this deposit reduces the pulp cavity in size. Sometimes in old age or as a result of pathologic changes, the pulp cavity may become partially or entirely obliterated (Fig. 1–5).

During the period of root development, the diameter of the root canal is greatest at the free or apical end of the root, at which level it presents a funnel-shaped opening (Figs. 1–1 and 10–5, 1). As the root continues to develop, this funnel-shaped opening is reduced in size, and finally, as the formative process nears completion, the opening becomes more constricted until at last the apex of the root is mature, with a small apical foramen or with small multiple foramina (Figs. 1–3 and 1–4).

Prolongations, or domes, in the roof of the pulp chamber correspond to the various cusps of the crown. The projections of pulp tissue occupying these spaces are called pulp horns (Fig. 1–3). If the cusp form of the crown of a tooth is well developed, the horns of the pulp chamber will correspond; however, if the cusps are small, the pulp horns will be short or missing entirely. In middle age and beyond, it is possible that posterior teeth might still have well-accented pulp horns (Fig. 2–7). When anterior teeth in young persons have well-marked developmental lobes, accented pulp horns may be expected, especially in the labial portions, as extensions into the three labial lobes. These are always more marked in young teeth, and they usually become smaller or disappear with advancing age (Figs. 1–1 and 1–5). Undoubtedly, in very young persons, a small pulp horn would represent the cingulum formation on anterior teeth and canines also, but in the examination of many tooth specimens over the years, the author has observed none with that horn demarcation. However, many of these teeth will show a definite swelling of the pulp chamber at the point of cingulum formation (Fig. 10–14, *A*, 7, 8).

The entire pulp cavity tends to become smaller with age, owing to the development of secondary deposit of dentin. Several things may contribute to this activity: malocclusion, thermal shock, occlusal trauma, and abrasion. Cross sections of teeth with substantial deposits of secondary dentin are easy to obtain. Often it is possible, when studying such sections, to see the original outline of the pulp chamber marked by the degree of translucency and color variation between the secondary dentin and the primary dentin (Fig. 1–5).

When studying teeth in cross section, it is most important to observe the labiolingual or buccolingual sections, for it is in these sections that the pulp cavities show the greatest number of variations. Students and even those in practice are apt to be less familiar with the root canal anatomy from the mesial and distal aspects. Routine radiographs of the teeth show the cross-sectional anatomy well from the labial and buccal aspects only (Fig. 1–6). Faciolingually, the dental anatomy is involved and complicated. The functional stresses that need most to be absorbed by the teeth are directed faciolingually; therefore, the anatomical form varies in order to withstand those forces. Anterior segments of the dental arches will brace themselves against forces brought to bear generally in a labiolingual direction. Posterior segments must withstand the greatest extent of functional force borne against them in a buccolingual direction.

The involved dental anatomy faciolingually will enclose corresponding pulp cavity anatomy. One must remember that the dental pulp is the original "tooth-forming organ"; the faciolingual form of the tooth is designed by the faciolingual mass of pulp tissue.

Unfortunately the cross-sectional anatomy faciolingually cannot be observed in radiographs when standard dental radiographic angulation technique is used. Yet, that information is of the utmost importance to the endodontist. Presently there is some research being conducted on the subject of dental radiographic angulation.[1] Often single-rooted teeth will have branching root canals or more than one canal. Teeth that are supposed to have one tapered root may present a bifurcation or apparent fusion of more than one root (Figs. 6–9 and 10–19). The clinician must be aware of the possibility of variations from the norm and must be continuously alert when diagnosing a case for endodontic treatment and for a probable prognosis. The radiographic examination may not provide all the necessary information, and therefore, one must rely upon an understanding of probabilities.

Figure 1–7 demonstrates the limitations that exist when radiographs are made with standard angulation (see also Fig. 1–8).

In the picture on the left (*A*) with the teeth in normal alignment the *maxillary second premolar* is in direct view, and the pulp canal appears normal for a young person; it is slender and straight. Also note the *mandibular left second premolar*. Now observe the picture on the right (*B*). Both second premolars are out of proper alignment, but the *maxillary* right premolar is turned 45 degrees, giving the outline of the pulp cavity as it would appear in a *faciolingual* section. The anatomy of tooth and pulp cavity differs completely from its counterpart on the other side of the mouth in proper alignment. The *mandibular right second premolar* is also turned enough to demonstrate rather well what the faciolingual dimensions of pulp and pulp cavity might be for that tooth. The *maxillary second premolar* above shows a massive carious lesion caused by the abnormal contact relationship. Undoubtedly the pulp is pathologically involved.

In Figure 1–8 the emphasis is still on faciolingual cross-sectional anatomy:

A. Observation of the *mandibular right first molar* (with the D.O. inlay) gives the impression that there are two narrow pulp canals, one in each of the molar roots.

B. This picture of the opposite side of the same mouth gives the same impression; the first mandibular molar on the left side has had successful endodontic treatment and displays two slender root canal fillings. However, look at *C*.

C. This radiograph was taken at an angle that failed to get a "90-degree" profile registration of the mesial root of the first molar. Here we see that the mesial root has two canals rather than just

[1]Walton, Richard E.: Endodontic radiographic techniques. Dental Radiography and Photography, Vol. 46, No. 3, 1973.

one, as shown in *B*. Later, when the permanent teeth are studied in detail, the mandibular first molar will be singled out as a tooth likely to present root canal variations in its mesial root.

A diagnostic approach to the manipulative treatment of pulp cavities must include the principles involved in gaining access to the pulp chambers. This subject will be covered in detail later when individual teeth are described; nevertheless, some mention of the subject should be made at this time.

Maximal exposure of the roof of the pulp chamber is advocated, so long as the tooth crown is not weakened in the process. Nothing is gained by trying to introduce canal instruments through miniature apertures. The discussions following this introductory chapter will explain why generous openings into tooth crowns are desirable.

In the meantime let us look at Figure 1–9, *A*. This is a drawing of a labiolingual cross section of an anterior maxillary tooth. Dotted lines indicate that a funnel-shaped opening has been made into the pulp chamber. A compromise has to be made in directing the approach. If the opening were made in line with the pulp canal of the single-rooted tooth, it could mean a reduction of the incisal ridge or cusp. Since the functional and cosmetic effect of the crown form is important, ridges and cusps must be left intact. The dotted lines in *A* show how the funnel-shaped opening can be made lingually and can be brought forward incisally as far as is necessary. It can be done without involving the incisal portion of the tooth. In the following chapters, a more graphic explanation of this situation will be offered.

Figure 1–9, *B* is a drawing of a buccolingual cross section of a maxillary molar. The dotted lines represent the design of the opening necessary for removal of the roof of the pulp chamber to allow for maximal exposure, leaving no undercuts and permitting sufficient angulation of instruments to achieve a "straight line" approach to root canals. Posteriorly, this means that the center portion of the occlusal surface, with its developmental grooves, is involved, the cut staying within the occlusal slope to cusp tips, and within marginal ridges mesially and distally.

Figure 1–10 shows the occlusal aspects of posterior teeth and the lingual aspects of anterior teeth in upper and lower jaws from the median line posteriorly to include the third molars. The outline markings in *A* and *B* represent the extent and locations of openings thought to be necessary for the approach to pulp chambers for endodontic treatment. Posterior teeth are to be opened occlusally as wide as would be consistent with good finish in the final restoration. Generous openings allow better reflection of light with the mouth mirror, thereby assisting the operator in locating pulp chambers and canals. Needless to say, the wider openings are also required in order to direct various points and instruments properly during treatment.

To repeat, the pulp chambers of anterior teeth are approached linguoincisally. The incisal margins of the openings must be extended incisally as far as possible without undermining the incisal ridges of the teeth. Because the incisal ridge of an anterior tooth is generally in line with the pulp canal, instruments should be inserted as nearly in line with the pulp canal as possible.

Figures 1–11 and 1–12 will be of interest when compared with Figure 1–10. They show the form of pulp chamber floors to be anticipated after proper access has been achieved. White markings suggest the approximate location of the root canal openings.

The plan of this Atlas is to review pulp cavity morphology and to show its relevance in clinical dentistry. Chapters that follow will describe the anatomy and the endodontic approach to individual permanent teeth. As mentioned previously, these chapters deal with specific teeth, singly or in pairs. The sequence of their consideration is governed by the indicators of practical experience; those presented first are the teeth most likely to require treatment.

The first molars are often the first victims of infection or accident because of their complicated crown form and their early appearance in the mouth before the child is mature enough to combat bacterial disease or to understand the rules of oral hygiene. Since there is little difference between maxillary and mandibular first molars, the maxillary first permanent molar has been selected arbitrarily to be evaluated first, in Chapter 2.

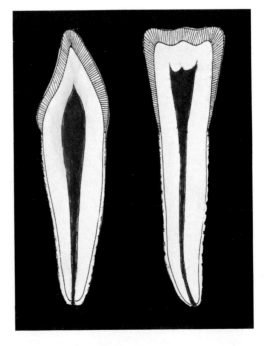

Figure 1–2 Drawings of lower anterior teeth that portray normal proportions. They indicate the similarity of form between the pulp cavity and the dentin body. Like comparisons may be made regardless of the tooth chosen for sectioning or the direction of the cut.

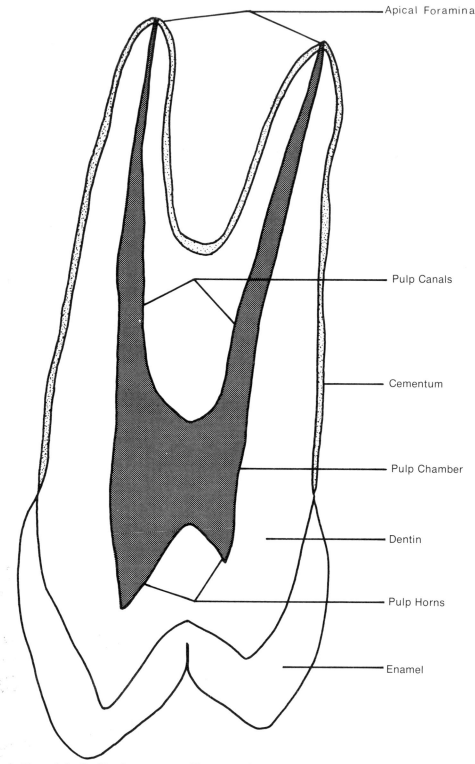

Apical Foramina

Pulp Canals

Cementum

Pulp Chamber

Dentin

Pulp Horns

Enamel

Figure 1-3 Profile of a young maxillary premolar in buccolingual cross section. This drawing was copied from an enlarged photomicrograph of an actual specimen. The silhouette of the pulp tissue represents the entire pulp cavity, which is divided into a pulp chamber with branching pulp canals. Pulp horns would be this prominent only in a very young person. (After Permar, Dorothy: Oral Embryology and Microscopic Anatomy, 5th ed. Philadelphia, Lea & Febiger, 1972.)

8

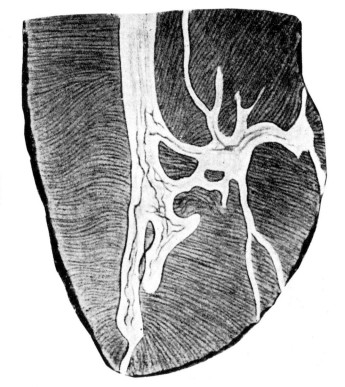

Figure 1–4 Apical end on root showing branching pulp canals. (Prepared by Dr. Richard H. Riethmüller.)

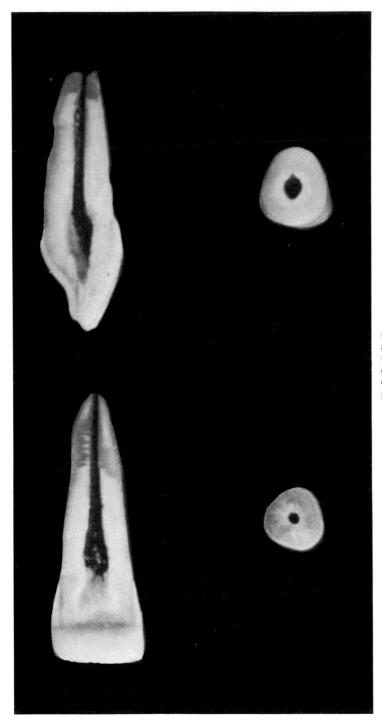

Figure 1–5 Labiolingual, mesiodistal, and root cross sections of a maxillary central incisor showing the differentiation between the density and color of secondary dentinal deposit and those of the primary dentin.

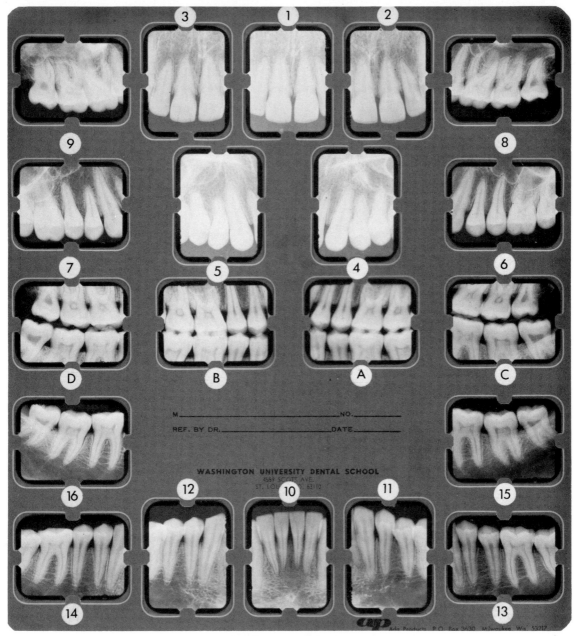

Figure 1–6 Complete dental radiograph examination.

Maxillary Teeth
1. Central incisors.
2. Right central and lateral incisors.
3. Left central and lateral incisors.
4. Right canine and premolars.
5. Left canine and premolars.
6. Right premolars and first molar.
7. Left premolars and first molar.
8. Right molars.
9. Left molars.

Mandibular Teeth
10. Central and lateral incisors.
11. Right canine and premolars.
12. Left canine and premolars.
13. Right premolars and first molar.
14. Left premolars and first molar.
15. Right molars.
16. Left molars.

Bitewing Radiographs

A. Right premolars, first and second molars.
B. Left premolars, first and second molars.
C. Right molars.
D. Left molars.

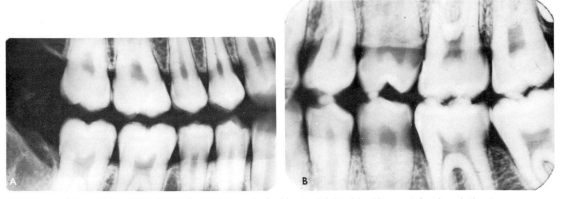

Figure 1–7 Bitewing radiographs. *A*, Left side. *B*, Right side. (See text for description.)

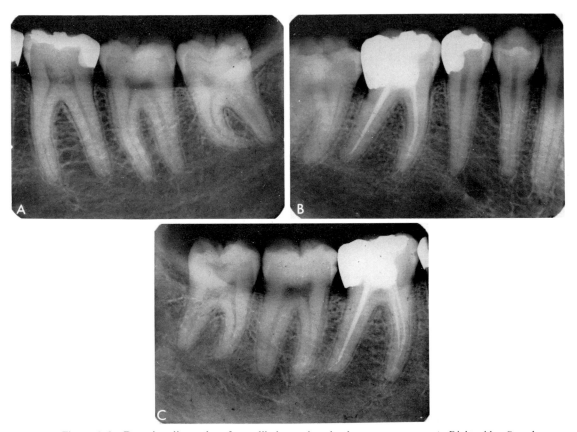

Figure 1–8 Dental radiographs of mandibular molars in the same person. *A*, Right side. *B* and *C*, Left side; note especially the canal fillings in the mandibular first molar. (See text for description.)

Figure 1–9 *A*, Drawing of a labiolingual cross section of a maxillary canine. Dotted lines represent the opening suggested for the approach to the pulp chamber. *B*, Drawing of a buccolingual cross section of a maxillary molar. Dotted lines represent the opening suggested for the approach to the roof of the pulp chamber.

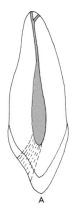
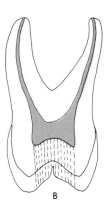

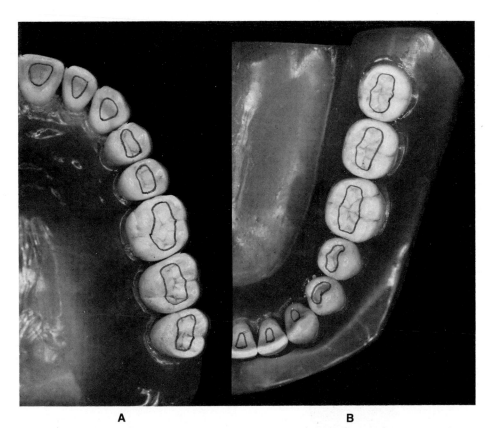

Figure 1–10 The occlusal aspects of posterior teeth and the lingual aspects of anterior teeth are shown for the upper and lower jaws left of the median line to include the third molars.

A and *B* show the outline markings of the recommended openings for the approach to the pulp chambers.

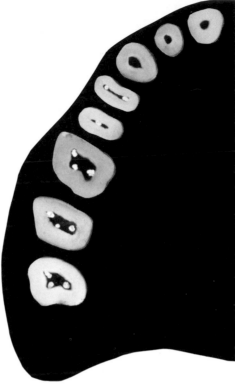

Figure 1-11 Cut-outs of photos of cervical cross sections of maxillary teeth. The cut-outs were carefully executed and placed in proper alignment on black background. Note the alignment and the relative shapes of pulp chambers. White dots indicate the approximate location of root canal openings in the pulp chambers of teeth expected to have more than one canal.

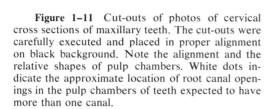

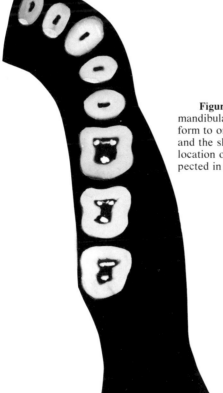

Figure 1-12 Cut-outs of photos of cervical cross sections of mandibular teeth. The cut-outs were placed in alignment to conform to one-half of the mandibular dental arch. Note the alignment and the shapes of pulp chambers. White dots indicate the probable location of root canals in the molars. Multiple canals are to be expected in mandibular molar roots only.

CHAPTER 2

Maxillary First Molar

In the macroscopic approach to diagnosis and manipulative prognosis in endodontics; it is always worthwhile to review the dental anatomy and to keep in mind the possibilities of involvement of the root form and of the complete pulp cavity form of any tooth that is to be treated.

Because records show that the first permanent molars are most often involved with pulp problems, even early in life, they will head the list for study. This chapter will confine itself to the *maxillary* first molar because records indicate that it may be the "number one trouble maker."

Volumetrically, the maxillary first molar is the largest of all the posterior teeth in the upper arch. Its three roots are relatively long and well formed. First molars seldom show malformation of crown or roots; this is not true, however, of maxillary second or maxillary third molars, the latter predominating in its frequency of variance. Another feature should be remembered in diagnosis and treatment: all first molars are older than other posterior teeth by 3 to 6 years or more, and the maturity of pulp cavities will vary accordingly. Occasionally in endodontics, the clinician is called upon to treat a maxillary permanent first molar in a child; therefore, it might be advisable to review the calcification table and to observe an illustration portraying the pulp cavity of the maxillary first molar from the age of 5 until the ninth or tenth year, when this tooth reaches maturity (Fig. 2–1). Successful endodontic treatment requires the development of sufficient root form for anchorage and at least the beginning of root end maturity.

CALCIFICATION OF THE MAXILLARY FIRST MOLAR

First evidence of calcification	At birth
Enamel completed	3 to 4 years
Eruption	6 years
Root completed	9 to 10 years

1   2   3   4   5

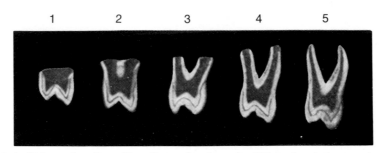

Figure 2–1 Pulp cavity of maxillary first molar, from the fifth to the ninth or tenth year. Lingual and mesiobuccal root canals are shown. See text for discussion. (From Broomell, I. Norman, and Fischelis, Philipp: Anatomy and Histology of the Mouth and Teeth, 6th ed. New York, P. Blakiston's & Company, 1923, Figure 141, p. 119. Used by permission of the McGraw-Hill Book Company.)

Figure 2–1 shows the development of the maxillary first molar in five stages as follows:

1. Approximate size and form of the pulp chamber at the fifth year.

2. The condition of the pulp cavity at age 6 or at time of eruption.

3. The change that has taken place at 7 years; the floor of the pulp chamber has been established.

4. A gradual reduction in the capacity of both the chamber and the canals. This represents the eighth year.

5. The size of the pulp chamber and the canals immediately upon maturation. The apical ends of roots have been calcified, establishing the apical foramina. Roots are completed during the ninth or tenth year.

In any review, a return to basic knowledge will require the repetition of details which may seem obvious. Nevertheless, without a review, the operator may overlook some aspects of dental anatomy that actually have only temporarily slipped his or her mind. Therefore, for the record, the characteristics of the roots of the maxillary first molar will be listed here.

ROOTS OF THE MAXILLARY FIRST PERMANENT MOLAR (Figs. 2–2 to 2–4)

There are three roots of generous proportions: the mesiobuccal, the distobuccal, and the lingual. These roots are well separated and well developed, and their placement gives this tooth maximal anchorage against forces that tend to unseat it. The roots' greatest spread is parallel to the line of the greatest force brought to bear against the crown; this force is exerted in a diagonal direction, buccolingually.

1. The lingual root is the longest; it is tapered and smoothly rounded but generously formed.

2. The mesiobuccal root is usually not as long as the lingual,

but it is broader buccolingually and shaped so that its resistance to torsion is greater. It has a broad, flat, and often fluted effect.

3. The distobuccal root is the smallest of the three, slender and smoothly rounded. It seems to be taking the place of the third leg of a "tripod." A profile lingual view of the tooth accents this root's angulation when compared with the other two roots (Figs. 2-2, *D*, and 2-29, *A*).

Because the form of the pulp cavities matches that of the crown and roots in miniature, endodontic procedures must be planned accordingly. A study of tooth sections will indicate the proper approach to pulp chambers and canals.

The maxillary first molar displays a pulp chamber that has a prominent roof formation structured to accommodate pulp horns (Figs. 2-7 and 2-23). This feature must be considered in operative procedures and when opening the crown occlusally for endodontic treatment. Care must be taken to ensure that the entire roof of the pulp chamber is removed so that no undercut remains to interfere with instrumentation or treatment (Fig. 2-16). Therefore, the first principle in endodontic treatment of any tooth is that proper access to the pulp chamber be made more than a minimal opening. Pulp treatment or instrumentation of the pulp cavities must not be inhibited by inadequate access. If the crown of the maxillary first molar is intact, the opening through the occlusal surface is made as generous as is consistent with good cavity preparation and finish in the final restoration (Fig. 2-8). The occlusal opening for the maxillary first molar will include the center portion of the occlusal surface with its developmental grooves; the cut remaining within the occlusal slopes to cusp tips and just within marginal ridges mesio-occlusally and disto-occlusally. If a large filling or carious cavity involves the crown, the occlusal approach for treatment must still allow for the minimal occlusal margin as described. Even though a wide disorganized opening into the crown of the tooth should be present, its shape might not favor the angulation and approach necessary for instrumentation in the treatment of root canals.

CROSS-SECTIONAL ANATOMY: DESIGN OF PULP CAVITIES (Fig. 2-5, *A, B, C, D, E*)

Buccolingual Cross Sections (Fig. 2-5, *A, D*)

Because the buccolingual section of the maxillary first permanent molar is of particular clinical interest in endodontic treatment, this cross section should be given special attention. As mentioned previously, the anatomical details of this cross section will not appear in standard dental radiographs. The buccolingual section will include a view of the pulp chamber and the mesiobuccal and lingual root canals, all in relation to the crown and root form of the molar. These root canals are to be featured in the study of dental anatomy

because they display characteristics that are particularly representative of the maxillary first molar and often differ entirely from a
survey of mesiodistal cross sections (Fig. 2–5, *B, E*).

The lingual root on cross section displays a long, relatively
generous root canal which corresponds to the generous proportions
of this root. Of the three root canals of this molar, the lingual root
canal will allow the greatest ease of access. Normally the canal is
rather straight and open. If curvature is present, it will not be
abrupt; the lingual canal is, of course, the longest of the three
canals in the maxillary first molar.

The mesiobuccal root, however, on buccolingual cross section,
stands out as a distinct anatomical variant (Figs. 2–22 and 2–23).
Endodontists are inclined to question whether instrumentation of
the mesiobuccal root is always successful. The complete removal
of pulp tissue is questionable at times, and the root canal can be
difficult to follow or enlarge, which would also handicap prophylac-
tic measures; all this in a tooth root having a distinct tendency to
present problems.

Buccolingual cross sections of 10 hand-picked specimens of
the maxillary permanent first molar can be seen in Figure 2–22.
Making an "educated guess," the author is of the opinion that approximately 50 per cent of the population's first molars will have a
single canal of some form in the wide mesiobuccal root. The other
50 per cent cannot be standardized with respect to the number of
canals, branches, or foramina that may be found (Figs. 2–19, *A,*
and 2–23).

These averages are based on years of practice and observation
as well as research, but it must be understood that they are empiri-
cal. However, there should be no doubt about the presence of
recognized variants in the anatomy of the mesiobuccal root of the
maxillary first molar, and the endodontist must be on the alert continuously when treating this root. More organized research remains
to be done in this field.

Mesiodistal Cross Sections (Fig. 2–5, *B, E*)

The mesiodistal sectioning of the maxillary first molar presents
the same view as that seen in the usual dental radiograph. It
includes the mesiobuccal and distobuccal roots. It might be noted
that this angulation will show a rather standard development for
this tooth. The radiographs will indicate whether roots are long or
short, curved or straight. Although the length and shape of roots
must be considered in endodontic treatment, there should be no
doubts concerning root form from this aspect because radiographic registration is dependable.

As demonstrated in Figure 2–10, pulp horns associated with

buccal cusps of the crown are prominent. From this angle (in Fig. 2–10), the rest of the pulp chamber looks constricted and deep as it opens into the respective buccal root canals. From the chamber, each root canal is angled sharply in relation to the chamber floor until midroot is approached (Figs. 2–11 and 2–12). From that point each canal dutifully adapts itself to the center of the root, whether straight or curved, continuing until the apex is reached. More mesiodistal sections of normal maxillary first molars that illustrate the foregoing statements describing the anatomy of the pulp cavity can be seen in Figure 2–13.

Cervical Cross Sections (Fig. 2–5, C)

By studying the cervical cross section of the maxillary first molar one can locate each root area in relation to the root trunk. Since each root canal is centered within each root, the survey will indicate the area in which each canal opening might be found in the floor of the pulp chamber (Fig. 2–29, A, B). The cervical section opens the pulp chamber, exposing the funnel-like entrances to the canals; normally, however, this open view is not provided in the nonsectioned tooth. Under operative conditions, the clinician must work through a comparatively narrow aperture in the occlusal surface of the molar. It is very helpful, therefore, to know the relationship of root to crown and the probable location of root canal openings in the pulp chamber floor.

The cervical cross section of the maxillary first molar can be described as being somewhat rhomboidal in shape, with the corners rounded (Fig. 2–14, B). The pulp chamber will be centered, and its outline form will reflect generally the form of the cervical section. The angles of the cervical cross section of this tooth may be described as follows: the mesiobuccal angle is acute and the distobuccal angle is obtuse, with both lingual angles conforming in general to right angles. This form reflects the functional form of the maxillary first molar when viewed from directly above the occlusal surface of the crown. The root canals have the following relationship to the pulp chamber floor: the lingual canal, which is the largest, will be centered lingually; the distobuccal canal will be near the obtuse angle of the pulp chamber; and last, but far from least, because it is difficult to locate, the mesiobuccal root canal will be *buccal* and *mesial* to the distobuccal canal in what seems to be an extreme corner postion, resting within the acute angle of the pulp chamber (Fig. 2–14, A, B). A map-like drawing showing canal openings and their locations with the connecting grooves in the floor of the pulp chamber may be said to suggest a distorted "Y," with the canal openings marking the ends of each of its extensions (Fig. 2–25, C).

DESIGN OF CANAL OPENINGS AND INSTRUMENTATION

The approach to root canals with root canal instruments (files, reamers, and the like) is favored by the smooth funnel-like openings in the pulp chamber floor (Figs. 2–15 and 3–9). The manipulation of root canal instruments will be handicapped if the chamber walls are scarred by careless technique, or if the smooth form of the openings that would be favorable to the operator are roughened in any way. A common error is careless opening into the pulp chamber, allowing burs (sharp-edged burs in particular) to create false markings in the pulp chamber (Fig. 2–16). Those who have encountered endodontic treatment problems can understand and appreciate the need for sensitive and careful procedure. A patient and deliberate approach to the work should be the rule. In operative and restorative dentistry, it is often possible to overcome a bit of carelessness by a change of plans in tooth preparation. The endodontist does not have this privilege; extreme care and slow, rather than rapid, advancement are necessary for satisfactory results.

The technique of manipulation of instruments for the purpose of cleaning and shaping pulp cavities and their root canals will not be discussed in this book. The mechanics of treatment procedures can be best understood in the clinic and in the laboratory where facilities favor a demonstrator and audience. As previously stated, the anatomy of pulp cavities and the diagnostic approach for manipulative treatment as they will be described here will provide the anatomical approach necessary for treatment planning.

PULP CHAMBER OPENING PROBLEMS

At this point, it might be appropriate to point out some common errors that serve to complicate instrumentation in endodontic treatment (Fig. 2–16). To repeat, deliberate planning and execution should be the rule in endodontic treatment, and this is especially true when nearing the pulp chamber during the opening of the occlusal surface of a maxillary first molar. The roof of the pulp chamber should be approached slowly with the bur and handpiece under control. If a sharp bur is allowed to fall into the chamber suddenly, the smooth surface of the pulp cavity will inevitably be marred. As the pulp chamber is approached, the bur being used as a drill should be exchanged for a round or "rose" bur. The floor of the pulp chamber with its funneled canal openings should be avoided entirely. Then, with pull strokes, the round bur can be used to remove all undercuts that remain in the roof of the pulp chamber, leaving a smooth, unscarred interior that will aid the operator in the location of canal entrances and in the process of pulp chamber cleansing.

One complication that may arise in pulp cavity treatment is the discovery of pulp chamber obstruction by secondary dentinal deposits (Figs. 2–17 and 2–18). Dental radiographs may indicate the extent of obstruction; nevertheless, the true state of affairs is usually discovered only after opening into the pulp chamber. In many cases a combination of deposits will be found. Secondary dentin will be deposited as a liner for pulp cavity walls, and pulp nodules or stones may be formed within the pulp itself (Fig. 3–1). Until such time as the two deposits join in completely obliterating the pulp chamber, the nodules can usually be scaled out. Fortunately, the latter situation happens quite often (Fig. 2–17).

SUMMARY – MAXILLARY FIRST MOLAR

The largest permanent maxillary tooth volumetrically, and the one that matures first in the maxillary arch, has three well-formed roots, no one of which resembles the others.

The mature formation of this tooth is typical and rarely anomalous.

There can be some variation in pulp cavity formation, especially that which involves the mesiobuccal root.

Macroscopically, variation from the single canal principle occurs least in lingual or distobuccal roots.

Lingual root canals are open, usually with generous formation.

Distobuccal root canals are small in diameter but are generally rather straight and accessible. The angulation in relation to the tooth crown can be extreme (Figs. 2–2, *D*, and 2–24, *B*).

Root canal instruments should approach canals from the occlusal aspect of the tooth crown, and the opening into the pulp chamber must be extensive enough to assist in treatment. A liberal opening occlusally facilitates the instrument approach to the floor of the pulp chamber and the the entrances of root canals.

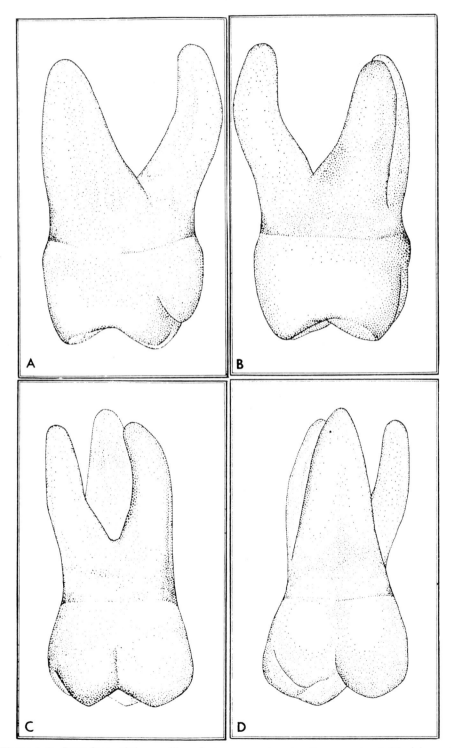

Figure 2–2   Root form of the maxillary first permanent molar, four aspects. *A*, Mesial aspect. *B*, Distal aspect. *C*, Buccal aspect. *D*, Lingual aspect. Note the rather extreme angle assumed by the disto-buccal root axis made evident from the lingual aspect. See Figure 2–24, *B*.

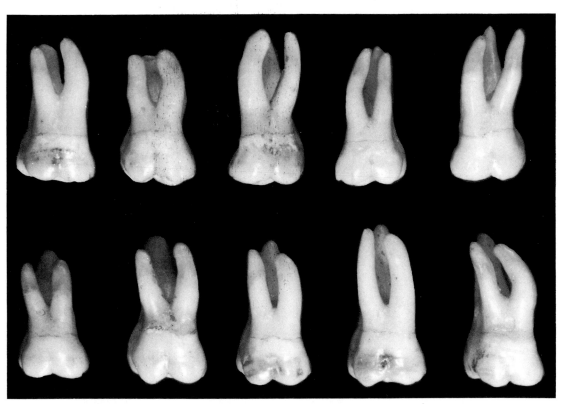

Figure 2–3 Maxillary first permanent molar, buccal aspect. These 10 specimens serve as a good representation of this tooth, with special emphasis on root form and development. The two buccal roots may be studied from this aspect. Comparisons should be made with mesiodistal cross sections (Figs. 2–9 to 2–13).

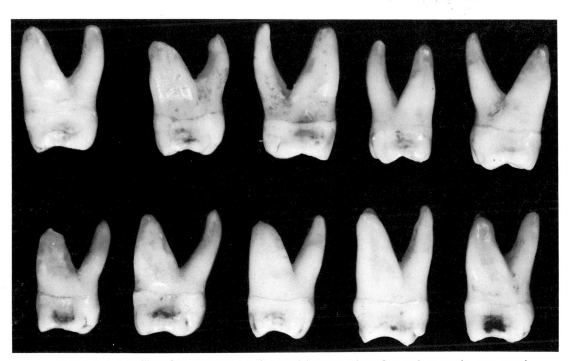

Figure 2–4 Maxillary first permanent molar, mesial aspect. These first molars are the same specimens shown in Figure 2–3. However, enlargement of the original photographs was not identical. A study of the roots from this angle emphasizes the unusual variance in form of the mesiobuccal root and the breadth of its root base when compared with the lingual root; the lingual root, however, is usually longer.

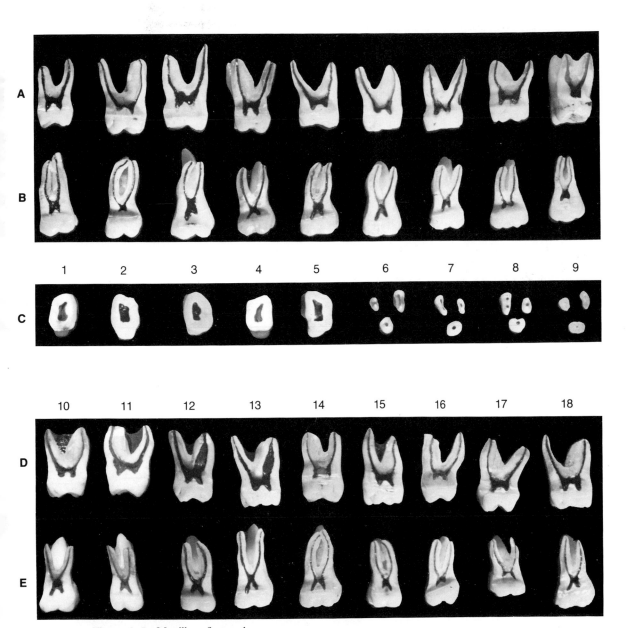

Figure 2–5 Maxillary first molar.

A, Buccolingual cross section, exposing the mesial or distal aspect of the pulp cavity. This aspect will not show on dental radiographs made in the usual manner.

B, Mesiodistal cross section, exposing the buccal or lingual aspect of the pulp cavity.

C, Five transverse cross sections at cervical line and four transverse sections at midroot.

D, Buccolingual cross section, exposing the mesial or distal aspect of the pulp cavity.

E, Mesiodistal cross section, exposing the buccal aspect of the pulp cavity.

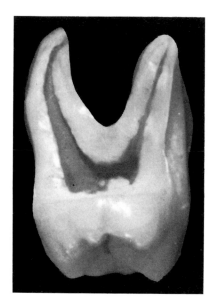

Figure 2–6   A cross section of a maxillary molar exposing the *distobuccal* root canal, in addition to the lingual root canal in a buccolingual section. After making a few of these sections it was decided not to demonstrate this cut in the records of cross sections of maxillary molars.

The mesial roots of all maxillary molars are the most complicated, whereas the distobuccal canal, although inclined toward constriction, is shorter, single, and nearly always quite straight. Also, it shows up quite well in the mesiodistal cross section. Exposing the single lingual canal from the distal instead of the buccal was of no consequence.

Figure 2–7 Pulp chamber roof of the maxillary first permanent molar. The crown of the tooth was severed at the cementoenamel junction buccally. The wax impression of the upper part of the pulp chamber demonstrates the pulp horn design as it existed in vivo. This illustration shows that the level of the tips of the pulp horns is inclined to be above the level of the gingiva if the gingiva is near the cervical line of the tooth.

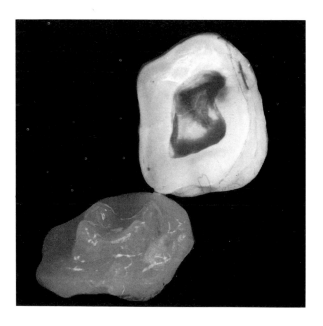

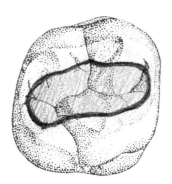

Figure 2–8 Maxillary first molar. Occlusal opening that is desirable for convenient access to root canals is shown. The cut will be centered in the occlusal surface, extending from the mesial marginal ridge to the distal marginal ridge, encompassing most of the occlusal developmental grooves; the opening is centered between cusps buccolingually.

1   2   3   4

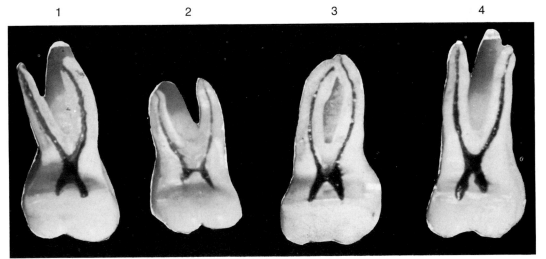

Figure 2–9 Four specimens of the maxillary first permanent molar, mesiodistal sections, show a similar development, but each also shows a slight variation when compared with the others.

1, Long, well-developed roots, but the mesiobuccal root and its canal exhibit more than average curvature.

2, Well developed, but the tooth with its roots is short.

3, This tooth varies from the average more than usual. Ordinarily, first molar buccal roots will spread apart. Both roots here are curved, long, and approaching each other apically. The buccal roots with their canals are curved. This arrangement is more common in maxillary second molar development.

4, This specimen has longer, straighter roots and canals than the average maxillary first molar. However, with all their variations, the four specimens have one thing in common: the angle at which the buccal root canals leave the floor of the pulp chamber (see Figs. 2–10 and 2–11).

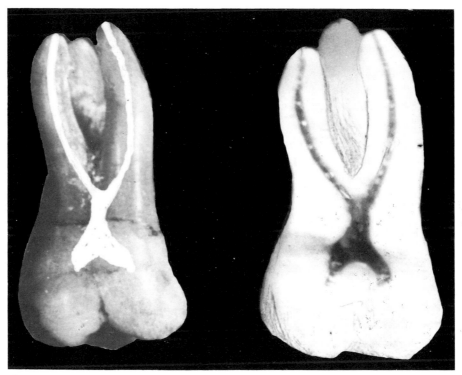

Figure 2-10 Maxillary first permanent molar—two similar specimens, one dissected mesiodistally, the other left intact. On the left, the pulp cavity, as exposed on the right, has been copied and painted on its side to show proportionate relations. Note the constriction of the pulp chamber floor and the proximity of the pulp chamber floor to the furcation of roots.

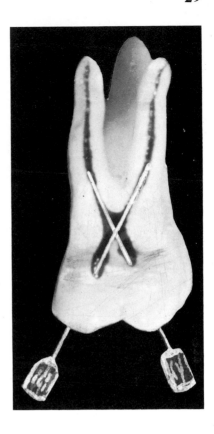

Figure 2–11 This illustration of a maxillary first molar with long, straight buccal roots provides a graphic picture of the angle at which canal instruments enter the two buccal roots from the pulp chamber floor. The simulated instrument handles show by their extension that a generous occlusal opening into the pulp chamber is required.

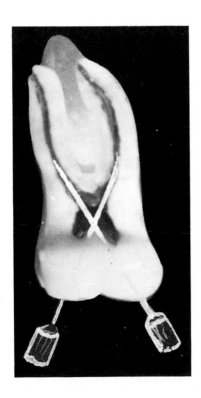

Figure 2–12 Maxillary first molar, mesiodistal cross section of the buccal roots. Simulated root canal instruments are positioned in the cervical portions of the root canals in the direction they must take to enter and to proceed. The variance in angulation is considerable, demonstrating the need for wide access through the occlusal surface of the crown. This specimen has roots and buccal canals with more curvature than that of Figure 2–11. However, the angles at which instruments enter the cervical third of the buccal canals are practically identical.

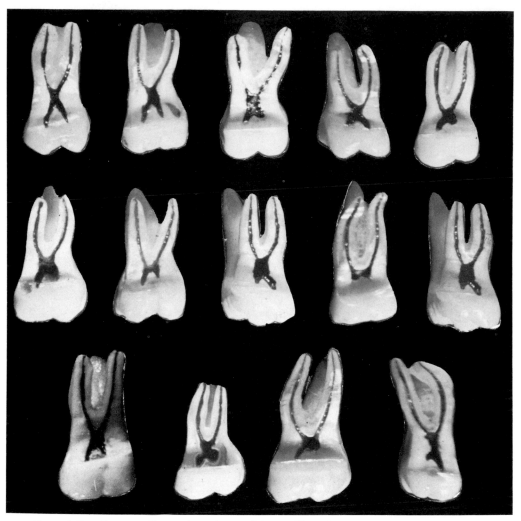

Figure 2–13 Fourteen dissected specimens of the maxillary first permanent molar, mesiodistal sections.

They may be recognized as being typical anatomically, differing only in comparative size and curvature of roots. Close observation will show that they seem to have one feature in common: the angle at which buccal canals must be entered as they leave the floor of the pulp chamber (see Figs. 2–10 to 2–12).

Figure 2–15 Maxillary first molar — idealized pulp cavity in a split ivory carving.

This carved model was intended for use in patient education. Close inspection of details in the photograph shows the carving's value when used as intended. The pulp chamber and root canals are larger and more ideal than usually found by the endodontist; nevertheless, they approximate the forms as they would appear in a young tooth at the time of root maturation. The illustration is placed here in order to emphasize the smooth continuous design of the pulp chamber, the pulp chamber floor, and the smooth funnel-like openings of the root canals as they leave the chamber floor.

Although this illustration is more ideal, in vivo the natural normal tooth will present smooth surfaces that will assist in endodontic treatment if those surfaces are properly preserved (see Fig. 2–16).

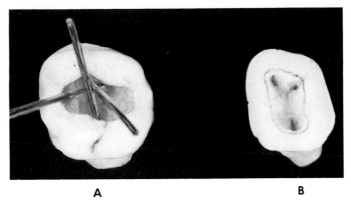

A   **B**

Figure 2–14   Maxillary first molar.

A, Occlusal opening suggested for proper access to pulp chamber. The probes placed in the cervical third of each of three canals show the variance of angle necessary for proper entry.

B, A cervical cross section of an upper left first molar with the cut made at the level of the cementoenamel junction. A typical first molar pulp chamber is exposed with three root canal openings on display in their accustomed relationships; they form a distorted "Y." The mesiobuccal canal takes a somewhat extreme position mesiobuccally because of the placement of the mesiobuccal root of the maxillary first molar; the distobuccal canal drops back distally and lingually, conforming to the placement of the distobuccal root; the lingual canal is centered lingually, directly in line with the lingual root.

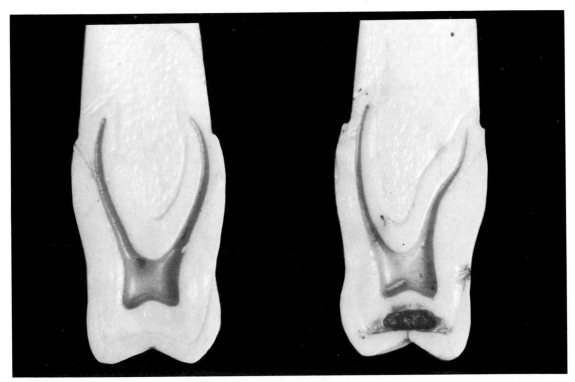

Figure 2–15   *See opposite page for legend.*

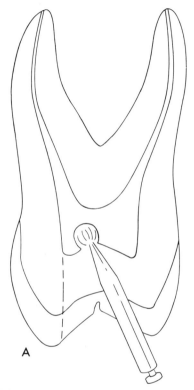
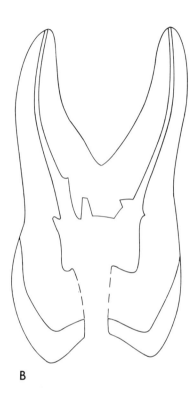

A   B

Figure 2-16 *A,* Diagrammatic illustration purporting to show penetration of the roof of the pulp chamber without marring any of the pulp chamber form. A round bur is to be used with a pull stroke to carefully cut away the roof of the pulp chamber, leaving no undercut which could interfere with the removal of tissue or with cleansing procedure. Note the smooth, curved surfaces of the pulp chamber and the smooth, funneled entrances to the root canals.

B, This illustration emphasizes the possibilities for disfigurement of the pulp chamber and canal entrances. This can happen when the operator makes an uncontrolled entrance through the roof of the chamber, and it most often happens when the occlusal opening is insufficient for satisfactory observation. Root canal instruments could "hang up" in any of the false cuts.

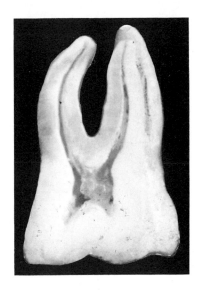

Figure 2–17 Mesiodistal cross section of maxillary first molar. A pulp stone is in view in the pulp chamber with a clear outline of the pulp cavity including the space for pulp horns. Note the peripheral deposit of dentin in the pulp horn spaces and in the floor of the pulp chamber. The pulp stone itself is usually formed within the body of the pulp tissue; therefore, if the deposit is not too extensive, the pulp stone will permit removal, more or less intact.

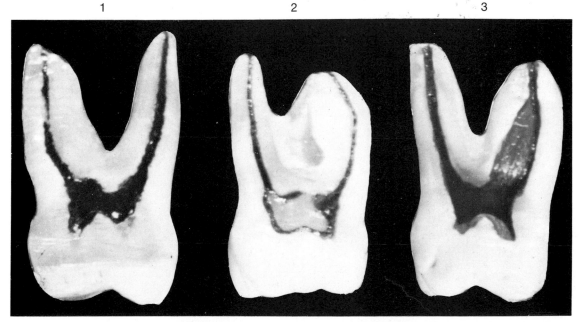

Figure 2–18 Buccolingual cross sections of upper molars, displaying pulp cavities.
1, Maxillary right first molar showing typical pulp cavity form.
2, Maxillary left second molar affording a splendid view of a pulp stone lodged in the pulp chamber.
3, Maxillary left first molar with a very wide canal in the mesiobuccal root.

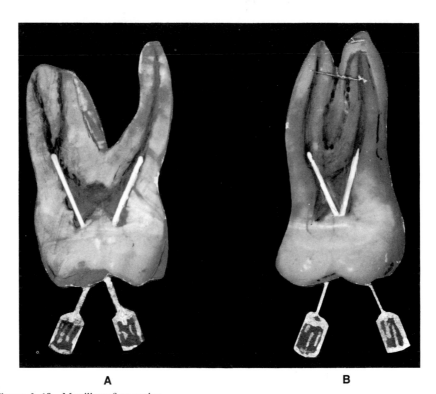

A   **B**

Figure 2–19 Maxillary first molar.

A, Buccolingual section. Simulated canal instruments have been inserted into the cervical portion of the mesiobuccal and lingual roots. Root canal development varies in mesiobuccal roots. This specimen shows a divided mesiobuccal canal in the middle third, ending in separate foramina. The lingual canal seems open with little curvature, which conforms to the average. It will be noted that the angulation of instruments for entrance into the cervical third of these two root canals differs considerably.

B, Mesiodistal section. This section was included in this figure to facilitate instant comparison between mesiodistal and buccolingual sections. There is a certain conformity in mesiodistal sections exposing pulp cavity design. For additional detail in instrument approach see Figures 2–12 and 2–20.

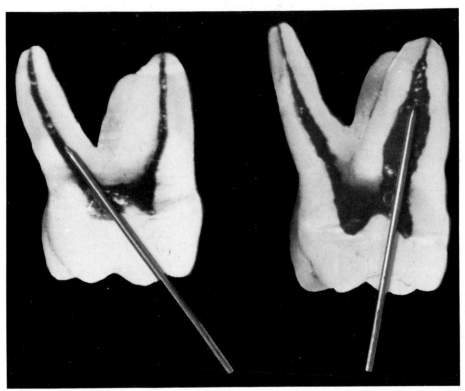

Figure 2–20 Buccolingual cross sections of maxillary first molars, featuring the mesiobuccal and lingual root canals. The angulation of root canal instruments varies considerably upon entrance to each root from this aspect. Note the variance in root canal anatomy when comparing the two mesiobuccal roots. The mesiobuccal root at right contains a wide, undivided root canal. Endodontic treatment of such formation is difficult.

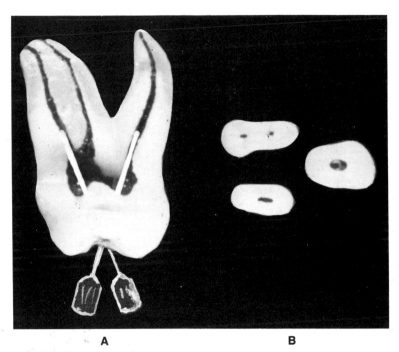

A   B

Figure 2–21 Maxillary first molar.

A, This specimen shows the mesiobuccal and the lingual roots sectioned in a buccolingual direction. Root canal formation varies often in the mesiobuccal root of this tooth; this specimen is no exception. In this case, twin canals with separate foramina are nearly parallel. Simulated canal instruments are pictured as entering the cervical third of buccal and lingual root canals. Although the directions of the two instruments are not in extreme cross purposes, there is considerable variation in the directional lines.

B, These midroot sections of the three roots of the maxillary first molar correspond to the specimen shown in *A.* The mesiobuccal root has two small canals; the distobuccal root has one; the lingual root has one canal which is somewhat larger and rounder than the distobuccal.

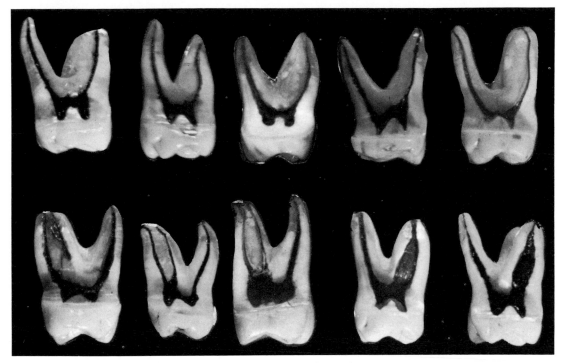

Figure 2–22 Buccolingual sections of the maxillary first molar.

The pulp chambers are exposed and the root canals as exhibited macroscopically are in view. In the upper row each tooth shows only one canal in the broad mesiobuccal root.

The lower row shows variations in canal design in the mesiobuccal roots, although these teeth demonstrate only a few of the variants possible in those roots comparable on cross section.

Figure 2–23 Two specimens prepared by Riethmüller about 1914. The paraffin root fillings demonstrate the spacing for a plexus of pulp tissue in each of the mesiobuccal roots. The tooth outlines represent the tooth form before it was dissolved away from the two root filling complexes. (Prepared by Richard H. Riethmüller.)

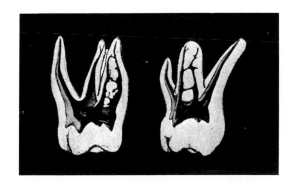

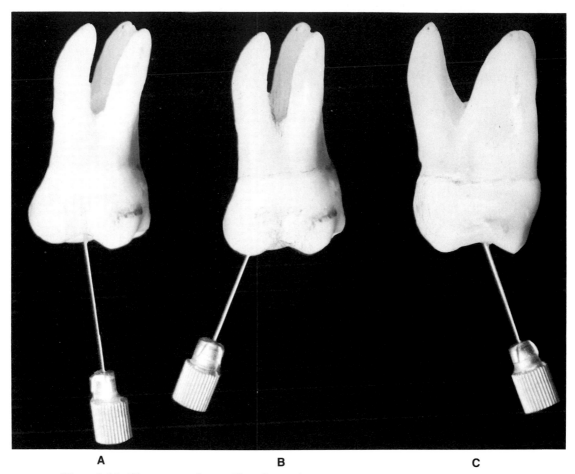

A   B   C

Figure 2–24   Three poses of a maxillary first molar.

A, Root canal instrument placed in the mesiobuccal root of a specimen tooth, showing the direction of entry in relation to the clinical crown of this particular tooth.

B, The instrument has entered the distobuccal root. Note the extreme angulation; this is the usual experience when working with the distobuccal root canal.

C, The instrument is placed in the lingual root; the view is from the mesial aspect. The rather extreme angulation is to be expected, a very different angulation from that of the other two root canals.

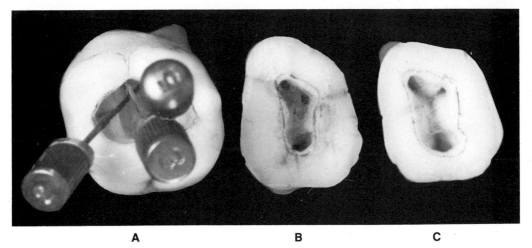

A   **B**   **C**

Figure 2–25 Occlusal aspect of maxillary first molars.

A, Three familiar root canal instruments are shown, one in each of the three root canals. The opening into the pulp chamber through the occlusal surface of the tooth crown follows proper extension rules.

B, Cervical cross section of one type of maxillary first molar, exposing the pulp chamber form and the location of the entrances to root canals in the pulp chamber floor.

C, Cervical cross section of another physical type of maxillary first molar, exposing the pulp chamber floor and the location of entrances to the three root canals.

Photographs like *B* and *C* are very difficult to make; artists' drawings may be helpful at times in registering details, but in order to understand true anatomical relationships, photographs of actual specimens are required.

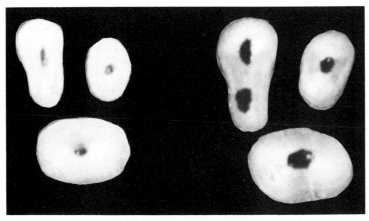

Figure 2–26 Midroot sections of the maxillary first molar.

The enlargement of the two specimens was uneven but the illustration serves well as a graphic comparison of two types.

The assembly on the left shows considerable calcification reducing the root canals in cross section but leaving them open enough to allow penetration.

On the right, all root canals in the subject displayed would be amenable to treatment, with two canals showing in the mesiobuccal root.

A discussion of macroscopic tooth form would be remiss if midroot cross-sectional anatomy was eliminated altogether. However, a practical approach to endodontic study gains little if much time is spent trying to analyze midroot sections. *More can be gained by locating midroot levels in a careful study of mesiodistal and faciolingual cross sections of the whole tooth* (Figs. 2–5, *C,* 6, 7, 8, 9 and *A, B, D, E*).

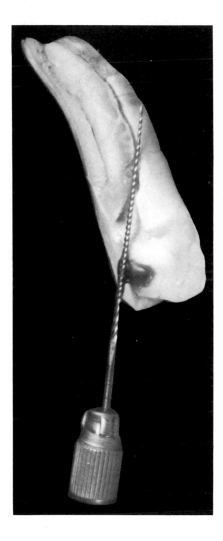

Figure 2–27 A sectional maxillary first molar specimen. This figure illustrates the need for a careful approach to a curved root canal with root canal instruments. An oversized file with some rigidity is placed at the angle necessary to enter the exposed sectioned canal from the pulp chamber. The illustration will emphasize the advisability of using small flexible instruments at first, in order to anticipate curvature. If a file or reamer is too rigid or is forced, it can scar the side of the root at the site of the curvature. This would make subsequent instrumentation difficult and could even result in a perforation in the side of the root if, for instance, motor handpiece instruments were later applied.

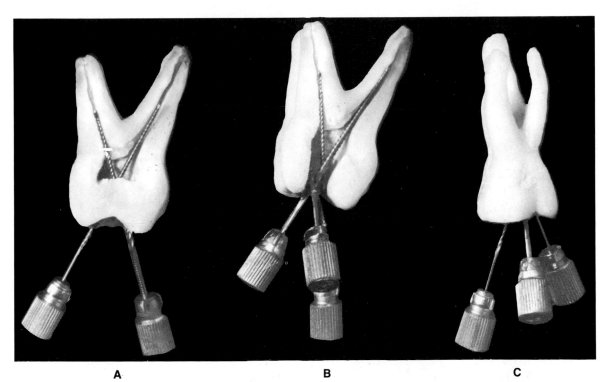

| **A** | **B** | **C** |

Figure 2–28 Maxillary first molar — *instrument approach to root canals.*

A, A cross section made buccolingually of the *distobuccal* and the *lingual* roots, exposing the pulp chamber from the side, but leaving the crown with its occlusal opening intact. The root canal files are placed through the occlusal opening in the directions necessary to follow the distobuccal and the lingual canals.

B, An odd angulation of the specimen in *A,* with the crown cut away to expose the occlusal opening of the crown, allowing full view of the pulp chamber. Canal files were placed in *all three canals.* This gives a perspective of the various angulations of root canal instruments as seen from a distal point of view.

C, A straight buccal view of the same specimen. The three instruments as placed in all three of the maxillary first molar canals give an added perspective for comparison of instrument angulations.

A   B

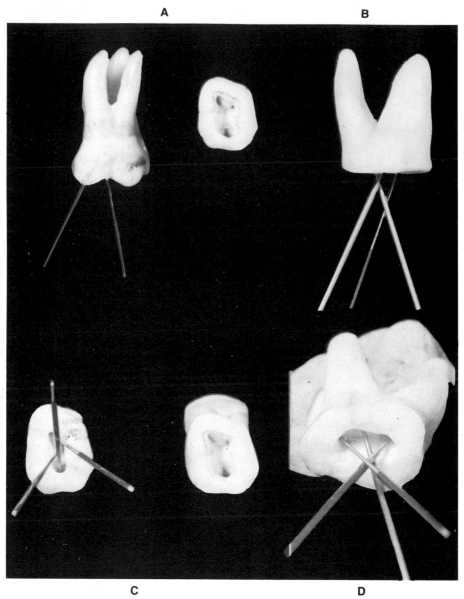

C   D

Figure 2–29   Four illustrations of maxillary first molar specimens. These should add perspective in a review of comments and figures recorded earlier in the chapter.

A, Buccal aspect of the maxillary first molar with instruments in the two buccal roots; alongside, a cervical cross section exhibiting the entrances of the three pulp canals in the floor of the pulp chamber.

B, The root portion of the cervical section shown in *A*, viewed from the mesial with canal probes placed in each one of the root canals. The variation in the angulation of probes is striking.

C, Here the specimen as seen in *B* is placed upright so the viewer can interpret the angulation of the probes from the occlusal aspect.

D, The cervical section exhibiting canal openings in the floor of a pulp chamber is placed on its mesial side and posed so that still another perspective is obtained; this emphasizes the placing of probes at cross purposes in the three root canals.

CHAPTER 3

Mandibular First Molar

Because the mandibular first permanent molar comes into use so early in life, it, like its counterpart in the upper jaw, is more subject to pathologic change than the other posterior teeth. Dental disease seems more likely to occur during the developmental period, beginning with the eruption of the first molars and ending when the adult stage is reached. Therefore, the mandibular first molar is discussed early in this text, since it may require endodontic treatment before most of the other teeth.

Volumetrically, the mandibular first molar normally measures largest of all the posterior teeth in the lower dental arch. Its *two roots* are relatively long and well formed. Although its total tooth form does not resemble that of the *maxillary* first molar, the lower molar, like the upper molar, has a similar biological function. They each set the pattern for the functional form of any molars distal to them.

Actual malformation is seldom found in mandibular first molars, but the age differential must be remembered when diagnosing pulp cavity formation, because there may be secondary deposition in many of them (Figs. 3–1, *B,* and 3–22, 1).

Endodontic treatment may demand familiarity with the age and tooth development of the patient in certain cases; therefore, a review of the chronology of development of this tooth follows.

DEVELOPMENT OF THE MANDIBULAR FIRST MOLAR

Figure 3–2, taken from the complete chart by Schour and Massler, shows the development of both first molars from ages 6 to 10 years. One notices that the mandibular first molar is a little ahead of the maxillary in the eruption process as well as in the maturation of root ends. Actually, according to the calcification table, the lower first molar could be expected to have closed root ends in a child only about 8 years old and should be treated accordingly. Apparently the child must reach age 10 before the endodontist can expect the same degree of maturation in the roots of the upper first molar.

CALCIFICATION OF THE MANDIBULAR FIRST MOLAR

First evidence of calcification	At birth
Enamel completed	2½ to 3 years
Eruption	6 to 7 years
Root completed	9 to 10 years

ROOTS OF THE MANDIBULAR FIRST MOLAR
(Figs. 3–3 to 3–5)

The study of pulp cavities requires a knowledge of tooth form and especially of root form. There are two roots of generous proportions: the mesial and the distal. The roots are well separated and well developed, and their form gives this tooth maximal anchorage when resisting forces that tend to unseat it. Although the mandibular first molar has only two roots as opposed to the three roots of its maxillary counterpart, the shape of the two roots with their anchorage in the dense bone of the lower jaw makes the lower tooth the more stable, as confirmed by attempts to remove this tooth with forceps (Figs. 3–10 to 3–12).

To repeat a principle described earlier, pulp cavities tend to copy the form of the crown and roots in miniature. Therefore, a study of cross sections will indicate the approach necessary to pulp chambers and canals.

The mandibular first molar possesses a pulp chamber, which, like the maxillary, has a roof formation that houses prominent horns (Fig. 3–8). If an opening through the occlusal surface of the crown is contemplated, the height and position of these horn formations must be kept in mind. If good access to pulp canals is planned, the entire roof of the pulp chamber should be removed, allowing no undercut to remain that might interfere with endodontic treatment (Figs. 1–9, *B*, and 2–16).

Pulp treatment or instrumentation of pulp cavities must not be inhibited by a lack of access through the occlusal surface of the crown. The mandibular first molar requires an occlusal opening as generous, with identical qualifications, as that of the maxillary first molar. There is, however, a slight change in relationship; while the *maxillary* tooth has the opening centered between buccal and lingual cusps, the *mandibular* molar opening is shifted a little to the buccal so as to be centered over the roots (Fig. 3–7). Buccal cusps of all mandibular posterior teeth are centered more over the root bases than those of the maxillary posterior teeth.

CROSS-SECTIONAL ANATOMY: DESIGN OF PULP CAVITIES (Fig. 3–6, *A, B, C, D, E*)

Buccolingual Cross Sections (Fig. 3–6, *A, D*)

The first molars biologically are forerunners of the other molars in the same jaw, and thereby serve as models in the formation of the latter teeth. A thorough study of the cross sections of the mandibular first molar, therefore, will give considerable insight into what may be expected when the mandibular second and third molars are to be studied.

The buccolingual cross section of the mandibular first molar will demonstrate a generous pulp chamber with accommodations for prominent pulp horns. Some of these pulp chambers are quite deep, the floor extending well down into the root formation (Fig. 3–27, *C*). The mesial root has the more complicated root canal arrangement of the two roots; thus, the cross section under consideration will show some variation in root canal design. Some teeth will have a single broad canal (although very thin mesiodistally), which remains quite wide buccolingually until it approaches the apical end of the root, where it narrows down to a pointed apical formation (Fig. 3–6, *A*, 3, 8). More than likely, most of the mandibular first molars will present two separate canals in the mesial root and many will join in a common opening apically (Fig. 3–6, *A*, 1, 2). Others will have the two canals separated all the way from the floor of the pulp chamber to the apical end of the root, keeping two separate apical foramina (Fig. 3–6, *A*, 4, 7, 9).

Mesiodistal Cross Section (Fig. 3–6, *B, E*)

The mesiodistal cross sections of the mandibular first molar present few variables in the form of pulp chamber or pulp canal. The pulp chamber will seem generous enough with the usual pulp horn formation, and the dual root formation will have the root canals centered throughout the root form. The mesial root will show considerable curvature in most cases (Fig. 3–13), the distal root appearing shorter and quite straight. Unfortunately, the longer curved mesial root contains the most constricted canal mesiodistally. The distal root usually presents a shorter, more open canal (Fig. 3–14).

Cervical Cross Section (Fig. 3–6, *C*)

The cervical cross section of the mandibular first molar is generally quadrilateral in form. Distally it tapers a little from the wider buccolingual measurement mesially. The pulp chamber outline reflects this formation in miniature. The pulp chamber floor can have two small funnel-shaped openings into the mesial root of this tooth, one buccal and one lingual. A single opening that is less constricted is centered distally in the pulp chamber leading into the distal root (Figs. 3–22 to 3–24).

Midroot Cross Section (Figs. 3–6, C, and 3–19, 3)

The midroot formation of the mandibular first molar is consistent with the major form of this tooth. Usually the mesial root will appear somewhat kidney-shaped, with two separate canals. Or it may show one narrow flat canal, the shape of the root remaining somewhat the same. The distal root is more rounded and should present one oval or flattened canal only (Fig. 3–28). Occasionally two narrow canals will be discovered in the distal root (Fig. 3–6, C, 6).

SUMMARY – MANDIBULAR FIRST MOLAR

The largest permanent mandibular tooth volumetrically, and the one to mature first, has two strong well-formed roots, shaped to afford excellent anchorage in the mandible: one mesial and one distal.

At maturity, the formation of the tooth is typical and rarely anomalous.

Macroscopically, variation from the single canal principle will be found most often in the mesial root. There seem to be three main variations in this design: (1) a broad canal buccolingually that is thin mesiodistally, pointing down to a single foramen apically; (2) a division at the pulp chamber floor into two canals, one buccal and one lingual, which seem to bend toward each other near the apical end of the root, ultimately joining to form a single foramen; and (3) a division into two canals at the pulp chamber floor, keeping themselves separate the entire length of the mesial root, each canal possessing its own apical foramen (Fig. 3–25).

Root canals in the distal root can be divided, of course, but most often they will be typical with single root canals buccolingually, and narrow or thin mesiodistally, pointing downward apically to a single opening at the root end (Fig. 3–29).

Mesial root canals may be the most constricted when compared with the distal canal, interfering with an instrument approach, whereas the distal root canal usually allows unrestricted entrance. In any event, if proper access to the pulp chamber is available, the angulation of the approach to the pulp canals with instruments is not extreme in the mandibular first molar. It differs from the maxillary first molar in this respect.

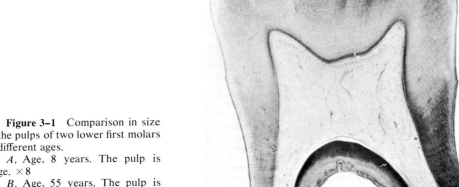

Figure 3–1 Comparison in size of the pulps of two lower first molars at different ages.

A, Age, 8 years. The pulp is large. ×8

B, Age, 55 years. The pulp is greatly reduced in size, and pulp stones (denticles) are present. The darkened area in the roof of the pulp chamber is representative of the secondary deposit of dentin. Also note the constriction of the mesial root canal. ×8 (From Kronfeld, Rudolph: Dental Histology and Comparative Dental Anatomy. Philadelphia, Lea & Febiger, 1937.)

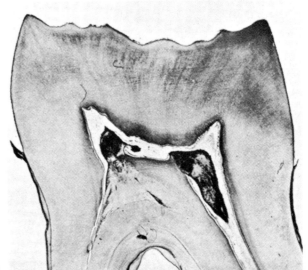

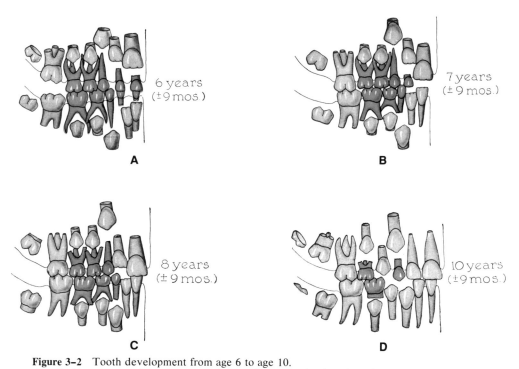

A   **B**

C   **D**

6 years (±9 mos.)

7 years (±9 mos.)

8 years (±9 mos.)

10 years (±9 mos.)

Figure 3–2   Tooth development from age 6 to age 10.
A to *D*, Four stages of development with special emphasis placed on the sequence of involvement of the first permanent molars, the mandibular first molar in particular. The deciduous (primary) teeth are shown in blue. (From The development of human dentition. J.A.D.A., *28*:1153–1160, 1941, by I. Schour and M. Massler, The University of Illinois College of Dentistry.)

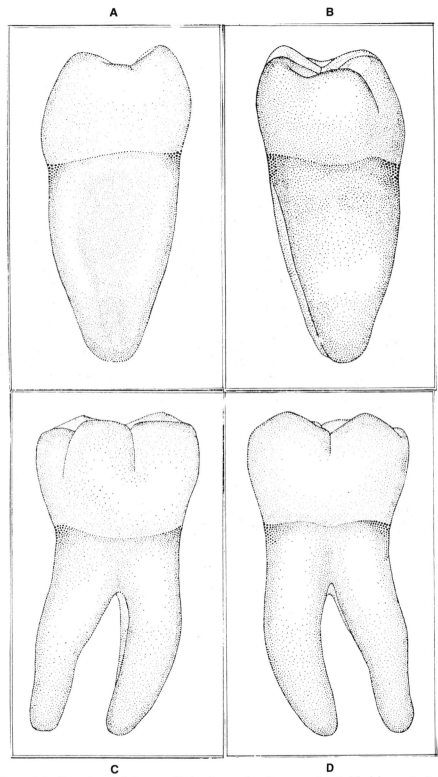

Figure 3–3 Root form of the mandibular first molar, four aspects. *A*, Mesial aspect. *B*, Distal aspect. *C*, Buccal aspect. *D*, Lingual aspect.

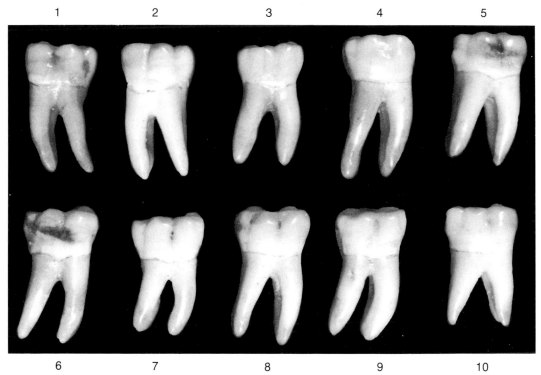

Figure 3–4 Mandibular first molar, buccal aspect. Ten choice specimens representative of this tooth, with special emphasis on root form and development. Note the tendency in most of them toward curvature in the mesial root as contrasted with rather straight distal roots. Both roots usually have distal inclinations. There is some variance in root length.

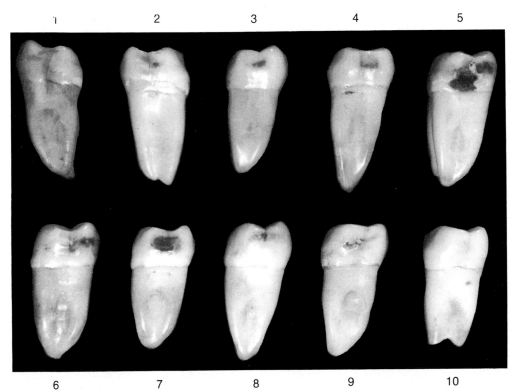

Figure 3–5 Mandibular first molar, mesial aspect. These are the same specimens shown in Figure 3–4. The mesial roots are very wide with developmental depressions centered the full length of the root. If one could see the other side of the root within the furcation, one would notice a parallel depression on the distal side (Fig. 3–11). Calibration of the center of the mesial root where concavities are superimposed is quite thin; the formation is similar to two roots fused in many cases (Fig. 3–10). An actual tendency toward bifurcation is not unusual (Fig. 3–5, 2 and 10).

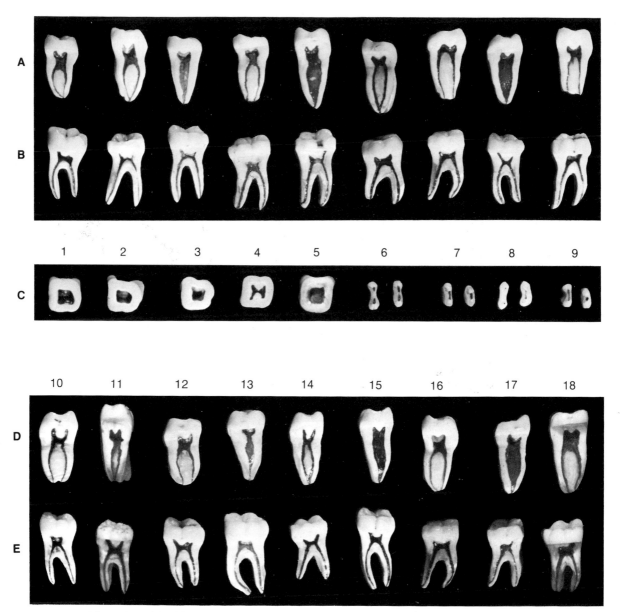

Figure 3–6 Mandibular first molar.

A, Buccolingual cross section, exposing the mesial or distal aspect of the pulp cavity. This aspect will not show in a dental radiograph.

B, Mesiodistal cross section, exposing the buccal or lingual aspect of the pulp cavity.

C, Five transverse cross sections at cervical line and four transverse sections at midroot. These are the openings to root canals that will be seen in the floor of the pulp chamber.

D, Buccolingual cross section, exposing the mesial or distal aspect of the pulp cavity.

E, Mesiodistal cross section, exposing the buccal or lingual aspect of the pulp cavity.

Figure 3-7 Mandibular first molar. The shaded area represents the occlusal opening that is desirable for convenient access to the pulp chamber and root canals; proper light reflection will be assisted also. The anatomy requires that the opening be placed buccally to dead center over the central fossa in order to be more directly over the pulp chamber. This is a variation from the technique required for the *maxillary* first molar.

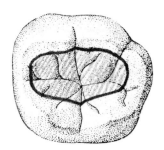

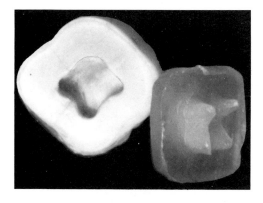

Figure 3-8 Pulp chamber roof, mandibular first molar. The crown of this tooth was severed at the cementoenamel junction buccally. The wax impression of the upper part of the pulp chamber demonstrates the pulp horn design as it existed in vivo. This illustration serves to show that the level of the tips of the pulp horns is inclined to be above the level of the gingiva if the gingiva is near the cervical line of the tooth.

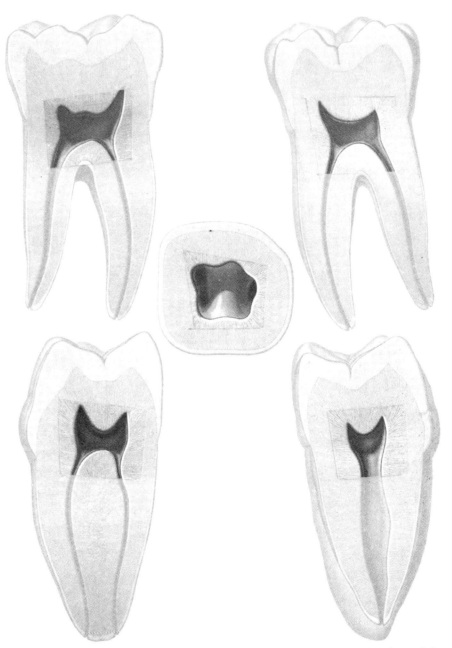

Figure 3–9 This excellent illustration purports to show the smooth, continuous form of the pulp chamber in a molar and the smooth, funnel-like openings into the root canals in the chamber floor. The illustration idealizes the situation somewhat; nevertheless, in vivo the natural normal tooth presents smooth surfaces that will assist in endodontic treatment if properly preserved. (Adapted from Zeisz, Robert C., and Nuckolls, James: Dental Anatomy. St. Louis, The C. V. Mosby Company, 1949.)

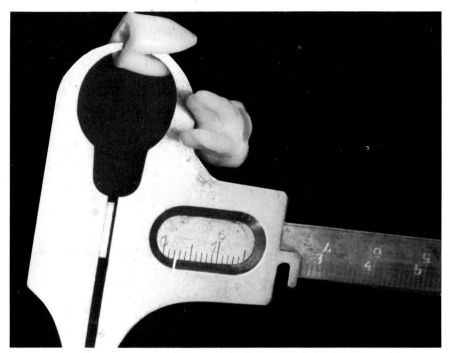

Figure 3–10   Additional perspective on pulp chamber and root form with unusual poses of two good examples of the mandibular first molar. The caliper beaks of the Boley gauge are measuring the thickness of tissue between the floor of the pulp chamber and the root furcation. The gauge indicates a thickness of a trifle more than 2 mm. Careless use of a high-speed dental engine drill could complicate matters here.

Alongside, a typical lower first molar is posed to indicate normal root formation when the tooth is viewed from the apical aspect. Both inner and outer fluting of both roots suggests "four" roots fused; indeed, the anchorage in the jaw produced by this formation is an approximation of that design.

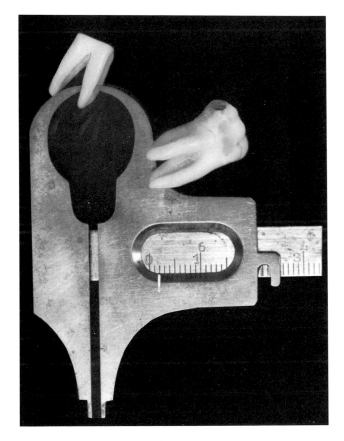

Figure 3–11 Here is an additional aspect of form of the specimens shown in Figures 3–10 and 3–12. The caliper beaks of the Boley gauge are placed in the deepest portions of the flutings on both sides of the mesial root about halfway between the bifurcation and the apex. The measurement is, in this case, 1.875 mm. This is in contrast to the 3.4 mm measurement at the widest portion (see also Fig. 3–19, 3).

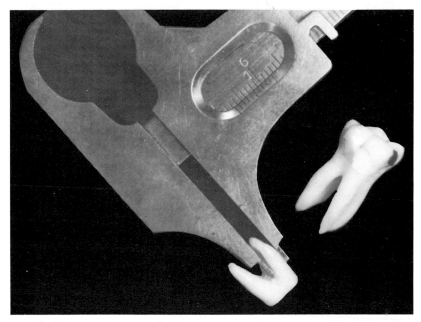

Figure 3–12 The same specimens in Figure 3–11 are shown here but are posed differently. The straight beaks of the Boley gauge are making a calibration of the widest portion of the mesial root of the mandibular first molar root section. It measured 3.4 mm in thickness. The root formation of the intact specimen may be observed at an angle mesiobuccally.

Figure 3–13 Mandibular first molar; two similar specimens, one dissected mesiodistally, the other left intact.

The intact specimen on the right has the pulp cavity painted on to show proportionate relations as demonstrated by the dissected specimen on the left. Characteristically this tooth features a rather shallow pulp chamber (when compared with the maxillary molar) and a thicker mass of hard tissue at the furcation site.

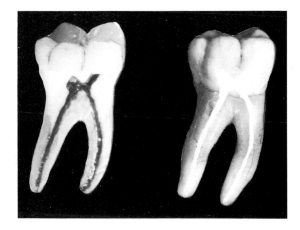

1   2   3

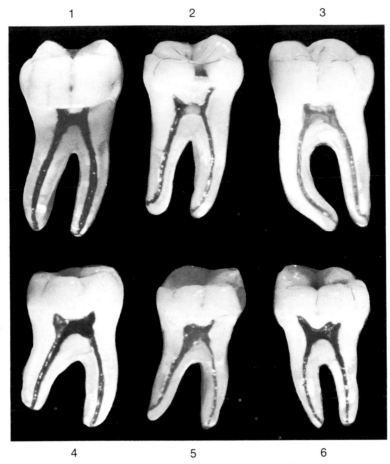

4   5   6

Figure 3–14 Six specimens of the mandibular first molar, mesiodistal sections. Although there is some variance when a comparison is made, at the same time there is a similarity of pulp cavity form. The specimens were picked to show tooth size and root form variations in teeth thought to have normal development.

1. A very fine specimen showing generous root canal and pulp chamber form. The shape of the mesial root is typical with a corresponding curved root canal; the distal root, although well formed, curves mesially at the apical portion more than most.

2. These roots are a trifle short, although well proportioned. The mesial root canal is quite curved; the distal canal, although typical generally in the center of a straight distal root, takes a sudden curve toward the apical end, making its exit on the distal side rather than at the root tip. This situation is not unusual. Note specimen 5.

3. This lower first molar is larger than average, with a mesial root which is longer and more curved than usual. The endodontic treatment would be made more difficult by root formation like this. Care must be used to avoid "hang-ups" of instruments or possibly even the opportunity for perforation if too much force were used. The pulp chamber and the distal root with its root canal seem normal. This canal has its apical foramen on the distal side of the root near the apical end. This root canal design is not a rarity; in fact three examples are shown here.

4. The tooth is well developed, but the distal root and its canal are short. The pulp chamber is generous, and the mesial root canal is centered in a normally shaped and curved mesial root.

5. Although this tooth is small, the roots, pulp chamber, and root canals are quite similar to specimen 2. The description of 2 is applicable to this one also.

6. The roots of this tooth are a little short for the crown size. In addition, the normal spread of the roots has been reduced. The pulp chamber has been displayed well in this specimen, however, emphasizing the tendency of mesial horns to have greater extension than others (see also 2).

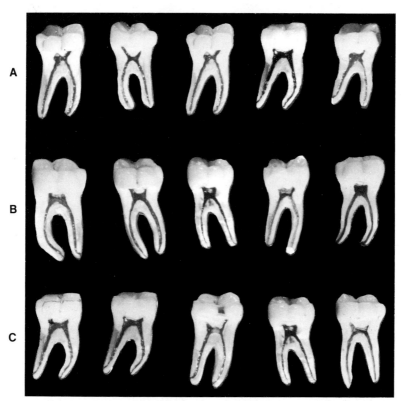

Figure 3–15   Fifteen dissected specimens of the mesiodistal sections of the mandibular first molar.
These specimens may be recognized as being typical anatomically. They differ mainly in tooth size and the length or curvature of roots; these features will, of course, affect pulp cavity design. In general, the design of these pulp chambers and pulp canals will reflect one common attribute: the angle of approach to root canals with instruments will be fairly constant for all from this aspect (Figs. 3–16 and 3–19). A lesser number will have broader pulp chambers from this angle, and these will allow the canals to be entered with a more perpendicular approach of instruments (see fourth specimen in *A* and first two specimens in *C*). Further penetration of instruments to root ends must take into consideration a characteristic of the lower first molar that is typical: usually the mesial root and canal are curved from the buccal aspect, whereas the distal root is is inclined to be straight. Both roots have a distal inclination in reference to the crown. Some mesial roots will be longer and more curved than others, and some of the distal roots will show variation in size and shape. The advantage from this aspect is that good radiographs can establish the situation quite accurately.

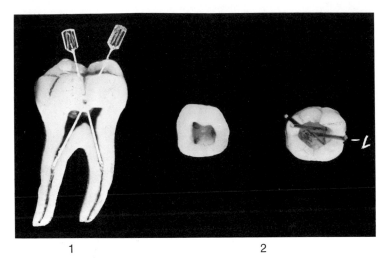

1   2

Figure 3–16   Mandibular first molars.

1. Mesiodistal cross section showing the buccal aspect of mesial and distal root canals in a lower *right* first molar. Simulated root canal instruments show the angulation necessary to penetrate the upper half of the canals. Careful manipulation will be necessary in order for the instruments to follow the curvature usually found in the apical half of the root canals, especially in the curved mesial root. Alongside, a cervical cross section of a *right* first molar exposes a pulp chamber floor with typical root canal entrances.

2. Cervical cross section of a mandibular *left* first molar shows the occlusal opening suggested for endodontic treatment. Probes placed in canal entrances demonstrate the varied angulation required for entry. The probe marked "L" is in the distal root canal. The other two have been placed in separate buccal and lingual openings of the mesial root.

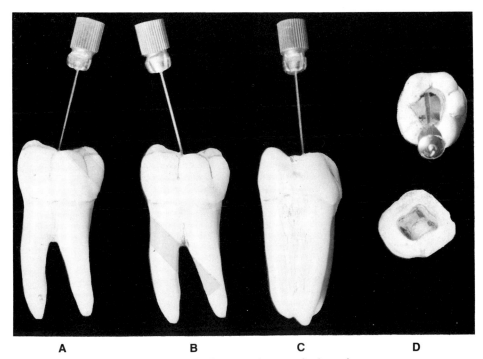

A   B   C   D

Figure 3–17   *See opposite page for legend.*

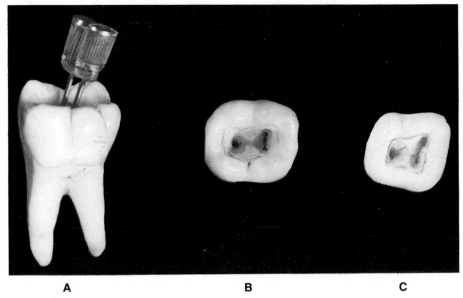

A   **B**   **C**

Figure 3–18   Mandibular left first molar.

A, Two pulp canal instruments placed in a natural specimen, showing the angulation and parallelism required in this case. The picture is typical.

B, The pulp chamber floor of another specimen as viewed through the suggested occlusal aperture. This specimen demonstrates the single, rounded type of distal root canal.

C, A cervical cross section of a first molar specimen that displays the same overall design of the chamber floor as specimen *B.* In this case, the openings to the mesial root canal are placed farther apart, probably indicating a separation of canals that are housed in a wide mesial root.

Figure 3–17   Mandibular first molar—some approaches to the pulp canals with instruments.

A, The instrument is placed in the mesial root; the handle has a distal inclination. Compare with *C.*

B, The instrument is placed in the distal root canal. The angulation is more extreme, leaning definitely toward the mesial. Because of the slant of the distal root, the angulation of the instrument often will be more extreme than in this example. Many times, mandibular first molars will have a long distal root, extending beyond the distal contours of the crown. In these cases, the instrument placed in the distal canal could approach the mesial marginal ridge of the occlusal surface of the crown before the distal root canal could be penetrated to its apex.

C, The direct mesial aspect of the tooth shown in *A,* with the same instrument placement. Here an inclination toward the lingual is obviously simultaneous. Compare the placement as viewed from the buccal aspect in *A* with the mesial aspect viewed in *C.*

D, Occlusal aspect of specimen and instrument shown in *B.* From this aspect, the angulation of the instrument seems more extreme, and the view of the pulp chamber floor is quite clear, aided by the wide occlusal opening. Below, a view at an angle of a cervical section of a lower first molar showing the floor of the pulp chamber. There are separate canal openings in the mesial root and a single broad opening distally.

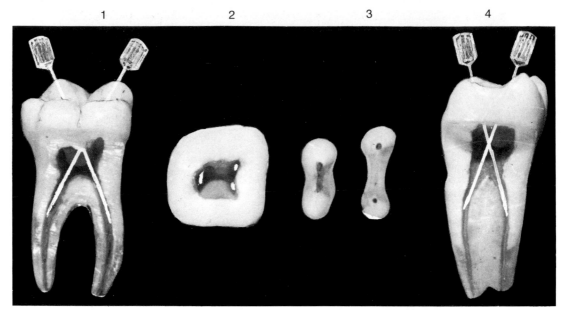

Figure 3–19 Mandibular first molar. This illustration shows the combined approach necessary to enter root canals when both mesiodistal and buccolingual cross-sectional designs are to be considered. The specimens pictured represent pulp cavity design commonly encountered in mandibular first molars.

1, Simulated root canal instruments in position at entrances to pulp canals, mesiodistal cross section. Note the extreme angulation necessary for insertion.

2, Cervical cross section; horizontal section at cementoenamel junction. White dots mark the approximate location of canal entrances.

3, Midroot sections for the type of first molar pictured. The mesial root has two widely separated round canals. The distal root is narrower buccolingually, with one elongated canal copying the shape of the root.

4, Simulated root canal instruments in position at the entrances of widely separated canals in the wide mesial root; the canals exposed by sectioning the root buccolingually. Here, too, the contrast in the angulation of the instruments is considerable, but less extreme than the angle necessary to approach canals mesiodistally.

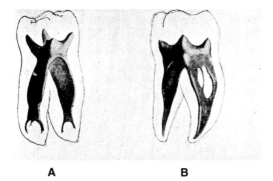

A   B

Figure 3–20 Two types of pulp cavities found in mandibular first molars.

A, This tooth possesses wide blunt roots. There will be a tendency to copy this form in the pulp canals within each root.

B, The root form of this tooth is more typical with pointed apical ends. Also, it has more variation in root width: the mesial root is wider and flatter than the distal root. The shape of the mesial root increases the possibility of root canal division, whereas the smaller tapered form of the distal root tends to confine the pulp tissue. (Prepared by Dr. Richard H. Riethmüller.)

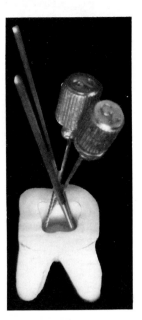

Figure 3–21 Cervical section of mandibular first molar with roots intact and four instruments placed in root canals. The files with handles show a contrast in angulation in the mesial root. The smooth probes placed in the distal root are closer together directionally.

1   2   3

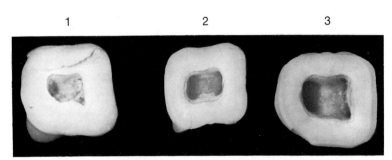

Figure 3–22 Three specimens of the mandibular first molar showing individualized situations.

1, When this specimen was sectioned at the cervical level, a constricted pulp chamber was found filled with secondary deposit. The extra material was blocking the root canals very effectively. Some loose material that had probably filled the pulp chamber formerly was lost in the preparation.

2, This lower first molar was smaller than average and very square in outline. The pulp chamber was shaped similarly, somewhat constricted in size, but the root canals were accessible.

3, This specimen of a large mandibular first molar is tapered more distally at the cervical level than considered average for this tooth (it is more like a mandibular second or third molar). As usual, the generous size and shape of the section are copied by the pulp chamber. Two accessible mesial canals are present, and one wide open root canal can be seen distally.

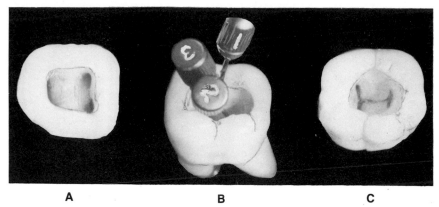

A   **B**   **C**

Figure 3–23   Another illustration of the approach to root canals in the mandibular first molar.

A, A cervical section made at the level of the cementoenamel junction. Note the apparent depth of the floor of the exposed pulp chamber below the junction level. This specimen exposes two separate openings to the mesial root. The distal opening is single and broad.

B, Root canal instruments placed in an intact lower *left* first molar with the occlusal opening made according to suggested specifications. Instruments 1 and 2 are placed in the mesial root. They are definitely not parallel in this case. Instrument 3 in the distal root canal demonstrates the usual angulation for entrance, thereby following the distal root alignment.

C, The general shape and location of the pulp canals are shown in this specimen of a mandibular left first molar. Dissection to open up the mesial root would probably show one broad but thin mesial canal (see Fig. 3–25, *C*).

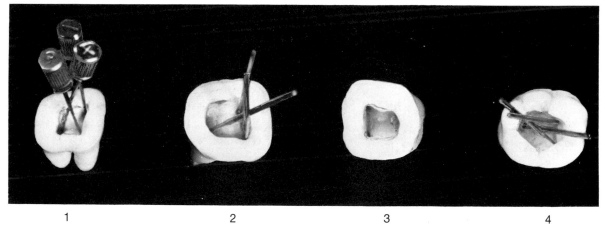

1   2   3   4

Figure 3–24   Four aspects of the mandibular first molar.

1, A view in perspective of a cervical cross section with the roots intact, with canal instruments in the root canals. Two of them in the mesial root seem rather straight and parallel with each other. The third instrument is angled considerably toward the mesial as it enters the distal root.

2, A view in perspective of the specimen shown in 1, but this time smooth probes were placed in the canals, thereby avoiding the obstruction of instrument handles in determining angulation. Now it is apparent that the probes in the mesial root canals are not quite parallel, and the probe in the distal canal seems to be positioned at a more extreme angle than seemed to be the case in specimen 1.

3, A demonstration of the floor of the pulp chamber in a natural specimen (cervical section) of the lower first molar. Mesial pulp canal openings are wide apart, and the distal opening seems single and wide. This is a typical arrangement. Note also the apparent depth of the pulp chamber below the cervical line of enamel of the crown of the tooth where the cut was made.

4, Another specimen (lower left first molar) with probes in the canals and the floor of the pulp chamber, showing considerable variation in the angles at which probes enter the mesial canal formation. Although the distal root canal is round and more constricted than many, the slant of the instrument mesially, above the crown is quite typical (Fig. 3–21).

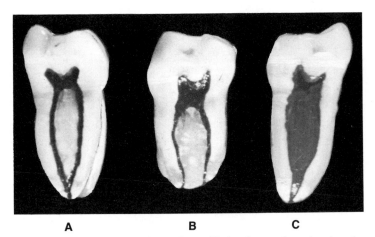

A **B** **C**

Figure 3–25 Buccolingual cross sections of mandibular first molars showing three typical root canal variations in the mesial root of this tooth.

A, This type is very common. Two separate root canals join near the root end to form a common foramen (Fig. 3–6, *A*, 1, 2).

B, This type is not rare, but neither is it a common occurrence. The pulp chamber is quite deep, and the two root canals remain separate with separate foramina (Fig. 3–6, *A*, 4, 7).

C, This specimen shows a pulp cavity mesially, which is a familiar type. The wide (buccolingually) and thin (mesiodistally) root canal, almost as wide buccolingually as the pulp chamber, narrows as it approaches the tip of the mesial root to form its apical foramen (see also Fig. 3–6, *A*, 5, 8).

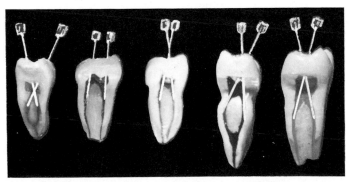

Figure 3–26 Demonstration of the necessary variations in the approach to root canals in different types of mesial roots. It will be noted that when these roots of mandibular first molars have a wide and blunt form, access with instruments is simplified. In other formations, especially those with "islands," the approach is more difficult.

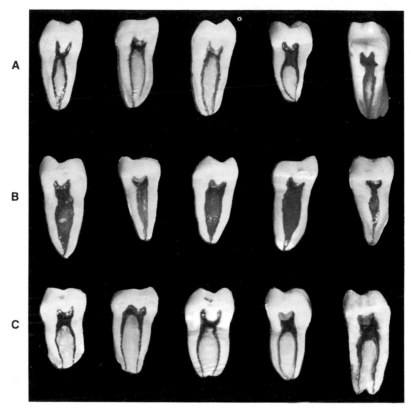

Figure 3–27 Buccolingual cross sections of the mandibular first molar. The pulp chambers are exposed and the root canals, as exhibited macroscopically in the mesial root, are in view. Generally, there are three types from this angle that may be found most often. They could be designated as types *A, B,* and *C.*

A, These five specimens have two canal openings in the mesial portion of the pulp chamber. Instruments will follow separated canals until an approach is made to the apical portion of the root. Here there is a tendency for the junction of the two canals to form or to nearly form a common apical foramen.

B, This group will have a thin, wide (buccolingually) root canal in the mesial root, often approximating the buccolingual width of the pulp chamber, and then continuing in this manner to the center division of the root length, where it begins to narrow as it conforms to the root outline. It ends abruptly at the root end in a single foramen.

C, These five specimens represent a type that is less ordinary than the other two, but a type to contend with nonetheless. The common characteristic is separate mesial canals in broad roots with separate and distinct apical foramina. Another feature has been noticed when analyzing the pulp chamber form of this type: often the chamber floor is at a lower level root-wise, indicating to the operator in endodontics that the pulp chamber is quite deep in relation to the occlusal surface of the tooth crown. The second specimen in this line does not conform to this pattern.

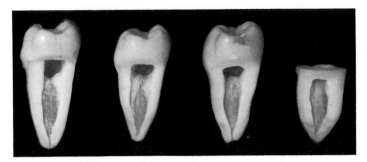

Figure 3–28 Four outstanding specimens of the mandibular first molar with distal root canals exposed.

This canal form can nearly always be expected to be present if the tooth has the usual well-formed root anatomy. In endodontic treatment, a misapprehension regarding this root canal must be avoided. Because it is usually open and accessible in the floor of the pulp chamber, the operator is inclined to think of it as being rounder and more generous in dimensions than the situation would warrant. Actually, it is broad in one direction only, buccolingually. Mesiodistally it is usually quite narrow and flat. It tapers suddenly near the apex in order to form a constricted canal apically (see Figs. 3–19, 3, and 3–29).

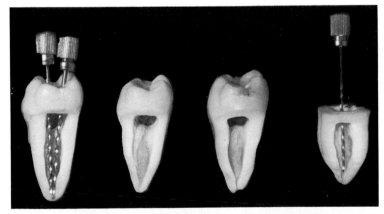

Figure 3–29 These are the same four specimens of mandibular first molars shown in Figure 3–28. Two of the specimens have had Kerr reamers size No. 5 placed in the distal root canals. Chances are that a reamer of that size would approach the walls of the canal mesiodistally, but the camera has registered a tremendous discrepancy buccolingually, even when two instruments are put in place. These proportional observations are to be kept in mind when the distal root of this tooth is involved in treatment.

CHAPTER 4

Maxillary Central and Lateral Incisors

Experience has shown that maxillary central and lateral incisors are often subject to damage by accident as well as by early carious infection. Therefore, maxillary central and lateral incisors will require endodontic care more often than most teeth, except of course the maxillary or mandibular first molars. Actuarial records certainly imply a greater frequency of accident involvement of upper anterior teeth, even though carious involvement is less likely when compared with the molars.

Being located in the front of the mouth, these teeth are liable to many kinds of accidents, especially during the years of eruption and maturation. At times they may be destroyed completely before endodontic treatment can be instituted. Even in severe cases though, roots maybe left intact, permitting restorative treatment.

A major problem is created when the pulp is involved and the calcification of root ends is incomplete. However, much excellent work has been done on this subject, both in organized research and by interested endodontic operators in practice.

DEVELOPMENT OF THE MAXILLARY CENTRAL AND LATERAL INCISORS

In Figure 3–2, in the preceding chapter describing mandibular first molars, four sections of the Schour-Massler chart illustrate graphically important stages in the calcification and development of the maxillary central and lateral incisors.

CALCIFICATION OF THE MAXILLARY CENTRAL INCISOR

First evidence of calcification	3 to 4	months
Enamel completed	4 to 5	years
Eruption	7 to 8	years
Root completed	10	years

Maxillary central incisors can have malformed roots. Although always generous on cross section at the crown and root juncture, the root may be abnormally short when compared to the crown length, the latter visible in the oral examination. Fortunately, standard dental radiographic technique will show the root formation. When dealing with the maxillary central incisor, one may not assume that the root length will be related directly to the crown length as found in most teeth (Fig. 4–3).

CALCIFICATION OF THE MAXILLARY LATERAL INCISOR

First evidence of calcification	1 year
Enamel completed	4 to 5 years
Eruption	8 to 9 years
Root completed	11 years

An interesting observation concerning these two incisors is that the small lateral incisor crown is often malformed with a normal root of considerable length, whereas the central incisor usually has a well-formed crown of generous size and a greater possibility of deformation of the root.

Maxillary lateral incisors may have long roots curved at the apical portion, but except for the few that are highly calcified with secondary deposit, the manipulation of instruments in most of them should be accomplished satisfactorily (Fig. 4–22).

OPENING INTO PULP CHAMBERS

The insertion and manipulation of root canal instruments in the endodontic treatment of maxillary anterior teeth is conducted through a linguoincisal opening (Figs. 4–11 and 4–13). Although the approach to the pulp cavity must be made lingual to the incisal ridge (the incisal ridge is directly in line with the root canal and root center), usually the single canals will allow the flexible instruments to be used fully (see also Fig. 4–22).

At this point a more complete description of the cross-sectional anatomy of the maxillary central and lateral incisors will be presented with appropriate illustrations. Some of the numbered figures on the following pages may not be referred to in the text. In such cases the descriptive legend attached to each one will be self-explanatory (see Fig. 4–14).

MAXILLARY CENTRAL INCISOR

CROSS-SECTIONAL ANATOMY: DESIGN OF PULP CAVITIES

Labiolingual Cross Section (Fig. 4–5, *A*)

The pulp cavity follows the general outline of the dentin body. The pulp chamber is pointed toward the incisal ridge and then swells with the increase in crown dimensions. From the cervical level of the crown it tapers gradually as it traverses the root, ending in a constriction at the apex. From this angle it may be noted that the pulp chamber portion is narrow and pointed, as mentioned (see also Fig. 4–7).

Mesiodistal Cross Section (Fig. 4–5, B)

The pulp chamber is wider from this view, conforming in general to the shape of the dentin body. It is not unusual to find definite vestigial indications of pulp horns in the incisal portion (Fig. 4–6, A, 1). The root canal tapers evenly along with the root toward its apex. As a rule the mesiodistal width of the root canal is somewhat greater than in the labiolingual dimension. Ordinarily the maxillary central incisor pulp cavity is not constricted; therefore, the penetration of root canal instruments is rarely difficult. The uniformity of the cavity makes it readily accessible, unless an unusual secondary deposit of dentin, which may include pulp stones, exists. However, a radiographic examination will expose the problem in that case (Fig. 4–5, B, 3) (see also Fig. 4–6, A, 6; B, 6).

Cervical Cross Section (Fig. 4–5, C)

The cervical cross section of any tooth is produced by cutting through the tooth at the cementoenamel junction, where the root and crown are joined. Usually this will expose the pulp chamber at its widest dimension and show the location of the root canal or canals.

This section of the maxillary central incisor shows the pulp chamber rather perfectly centered (Fig. 4–5, C). In young individuals, the chamber and canal will be "roundly triangular" in outline, which, in this instance, reflects the root outline most typical of the tooth. In older individuals, the pulp cavity at this level becomes round or crescent-shaped, influenced by secondary dentinal deposit as age advances (Fig. 4–5, C, 4). Although the typical cervical cross section of this tooth will be triangular with rounded corners, some maxillary central incisors present a different picture. They will look rectangular generally or square with rounded corners (Fig. 4–5, C, 1). The calibration will be generous all around. This bulk provides the crown with the substantial base it requires.

MAXILLARY LATERAL INCISOR

CROSS-SECTIONAL ANATOMY: DESIGN OF PULP CAVITIES

Labiolingual Cross Section (Fig. 4–18, A)

The anatomical form of the pulp cavity of the maxillary lateral incisor resembles that of the central incisor because the two teeth have a similar functional form (Fig. 4–17). Dimensionally, the lateral incisor is smaller except for root length. Often the root of the lateral will prove to be the longer of the two. The description of the maxillary central incisor pulp cavity, when viewing this cross section, may be applied to the lateral incisor (compare with Fig. 4–5).

Mesiodistal Cross Section (Fig. 4–18, *B*)

The pulp cavity displayed by this section conforms generally to the outline of the dentin body of the tooth. It will be narrower overall than that found in the maxillary central incisor because of the smaller dimensions of the lateral incisor. However, the root canal is not constricted as a rule, which favors root treatment. There is one distinction when comparing this tooth to the maxillary central incisor; the pulp chamber of the maxillary lateral will usually show a rounded form incisally, seldom showing evidences of a design to accommodate pulp horns (compare Fig. 4–18, *B*, with Fig. 4–5, *B*).

Cervical Cross Section

The cervical cross section shows the pulp chamber and single canal well centered. Since the anatomy of the lateral incisor shows considerable variation, the shape of the canal will vary also. Some of the specimens displayed in Figure 4–18, *C* show considerable secondary dentin constriction.

SUMMARY – MAXILLARY CENTRAL AND LATERAL INCISORS

Maxillary central and lateral incisors are subject to fracture by accident, especially during elementary and high school years; contact sports and industrial accidents also play a part. Endodontic care can often assist in preventing dental losses in the anterior area of the mouth regardless of the cause of pulp involvement.

These central and lateral incisors have straight and accessible pulp cavities, offering little resistance to instrumentation. The open root canals, in the central incisors particularly, tend to have more open apical foramina also. Therefore, care must be observed during instrumentation in order to avoid unnecessary tissue damage apically.

The central incisors may have short roots compared to their crown length. Except for this possibility, maxillary central incisors rarely show deformity.

The lateral incisors are frequently anomalous, with dwarfed or misshapen crowns rather than roots. Root canals are usually accessible without abrupt curvature even though some curvature might be encountered apically (Figs. 4–22 and 4–21).

In gaining access through the lingual surface of the crown for the introduction of instruments, a positive technique must be observed in order to overcome anatomical difficulties. Both incisors require a careful approach (Figs. 4–13 and 4–22).

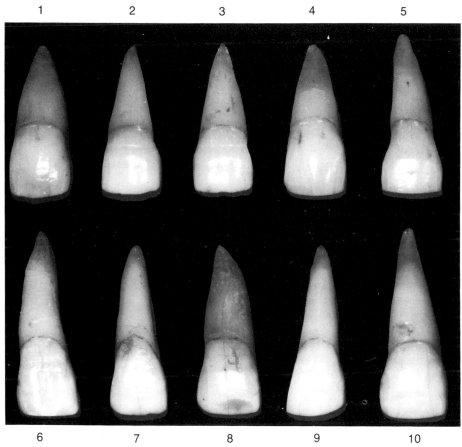

Figure 4–1 Maxillary central incisor—root form, labial aspect. These 10 specimens serve as good representatives of this tooth with special emphasis placed on root form and development. The roots have bulk and are evenly tapered; however, in endodontic diagnosis one must be aware of a possibility which is not apparent in this illustration—central incisors sometimes have short roots compared to crown length (Fig. 4–3). Maxillary central incisor crowns are seldom malformed.

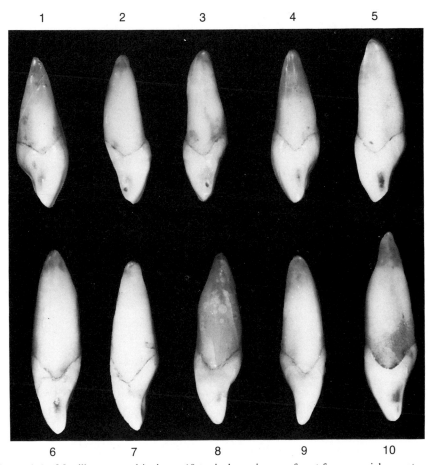

Figure 4–2 Maxillary central incisor—10 typical specimens of root form, mesial aspect.
Normal root length should be about one and one-third the crown length. The specimens here show-ing normal maxillary central incisor roots should be associated with the figures in this chapter that show the cross-sectional design of pulp cavities (Figs. 4–5 to 4–7).

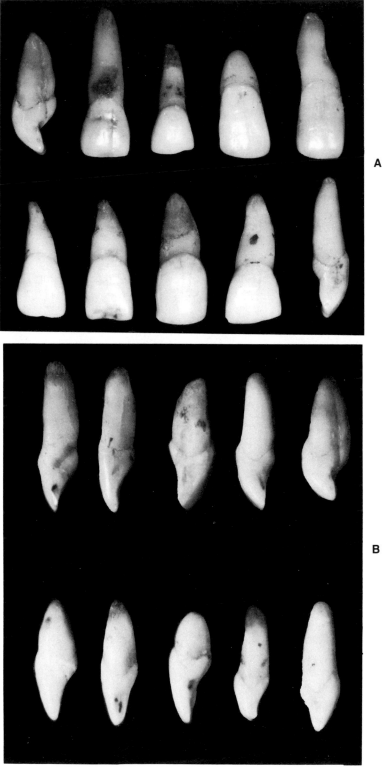

Figure 4–3   *See opposite page for legend.*

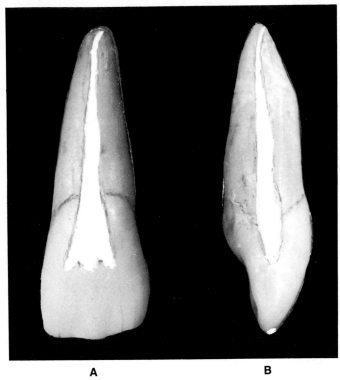

A   **B**

Figure 4–4 Maxillary central incisor. *A*, Labial aspect. *B*, Distal aspect.

Normal pulp cavity forms are painted on the surfaces as they might be seen normally in cross sections (see Figs. 4–6 and 4–7). Note the comparison between the spacing and form of the pulp chamber portion in the crown of one aspect as distinguished from the other. Viewed from the mesial or distal aspect the pulp chamber will be quite narrow labiolingually, and it will appear to be pointed incisally.

Figure 4–3 Maxillary central incisor—crown and root variations.

A, An assembly of 10 specimens showing anatomical variations in crown versus root design. Those with roots abnormally short are of interest in endodontics because they occur often and must be looked for.

B, Ten specimens showing anatomical variations as viewed from the mesial aspect. Some of these are shown in *A*. The "hawk-bill" types of tooth crowns (upper right) complicate the linguoincisal approach to pulp cavities.

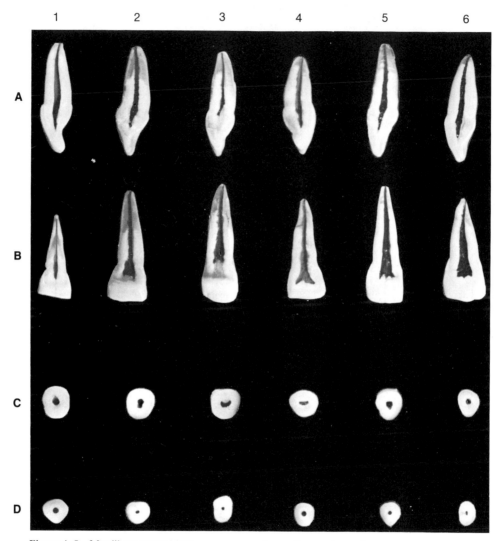

Figure 4–5   Maxillary central incisor—cross sections of natural specimens.
A, 1 to 6, Labiolingual sections. This aspect does not show in radiographs taken the standard way.
B, 1 to 6, Mesiodistal sections.
C, 1 to 6, Cervical sections of root.
D, 1 to 6, Midroot sections.

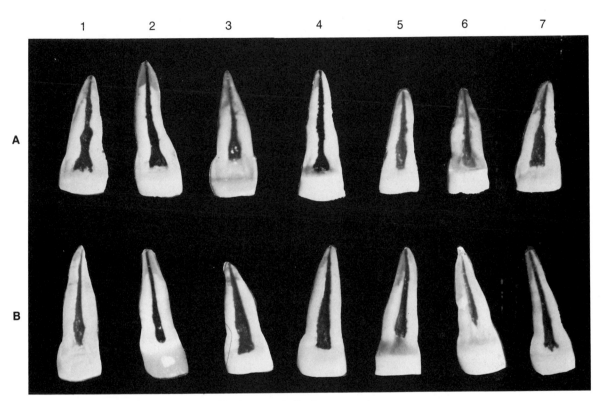

Figure 4–6 Maxillary central incisor, mesiodistal cross sections.

Because the crowns and roots of these teeth are relatively broad, normally the pulp cavities are wide and accessible; they are wider from this aspect than from the labiolingual aspect (Fig. 4–7). No problems involving entry are associated with the latter aspect because the root has generous proportions labiolingually.

Close inspection of individual specimens in this figure will be interesting: 1 and 5 (*A*) have cavities that are unevenly tapered; in 3 and 6 (*A*) and 5 and 6 (*B*) pulp chamber portions are obliterated by secondary deposit; 1 and 4 (*A*) and 7 (*B*) have retained spaces for pulp horns.

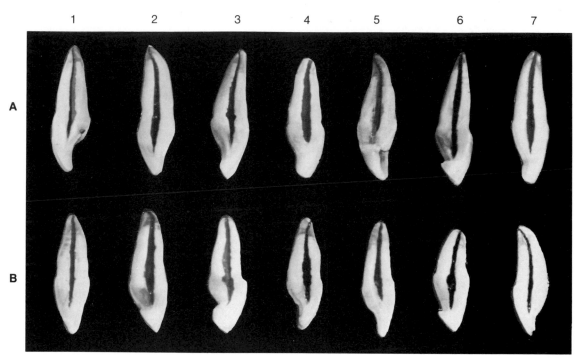

Figure 4–7 Maxillary central incisor, labiolingual cross sections. The essential form of the pulp cavities from this aspect, when compared with the mesiodistal cross sections in Figure 4–6, shows this variation; the cavities seem to be more slender throughout, more evenly tapered from this aspect, with the pulp chamber portions pointing narrowly toward the incisal ridges. Another interesting observation: from this view it is surprising how often the root canal will take a turn in a labial direction as it approaches the apical end of the root (*A* 2, 5, 7; *B*, 4, 7). This curvature does not show on radiographs taken in the usual manner.

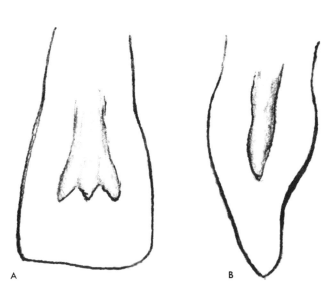

Figure 4–8 A rendition of pulp tissue within tooth outlines. The shaded area has three-dimensional quality which helps to emphasize the actual form of the soft tissue to be found in the pulp cavities. Empty cavities in cross sections may lack the emphasis necessary to create proper perspective.

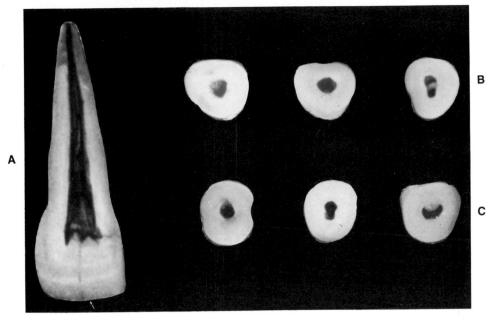

Figure 4–9 Maxillary central incisor.

A, Mesiodistal cross section of a tooth specimen showing a pulp cavity of generous proportions. Note the definite pulp horn projections in the pulp chamber division. There is no demarcation between pulp chamber and pulp canal in single-rooted teeth; technically there is a pulp chamber roof but no pulp chamber floor because the two portions of the pulp cavity are combined and continuous.

B, Three cervical cross sections made at the juncture of crown and root. These are perhaps most typical in outline form, being "roundly triangular." The pulp cavity space represents the "floor" of the pulp chamber.

C, Three additional cervical cross sections of maxillary central incisors represent another outline form of the root trunk often found. This type has a "rounded square" appearance.

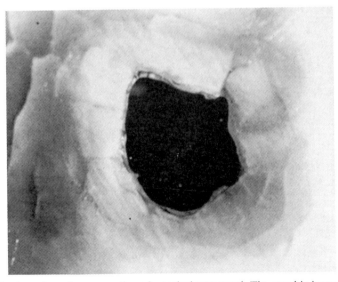

Figure 4–10 An enlarged cross section of a typical root canal. The canal is irregular in shape with frequent ramifications into the dentin, as seen in the upper right. This demonstrates very clearly the need for enlargement and reshaping in order to facilitate proper filling and sealing of the root canal. (From Sommer, R. F., Ostrander, F. D., and Crowley, M. C.: Clinical Endodontics, 3rd ed. Philadelphia, W. B. Saunders Co., 1956.)

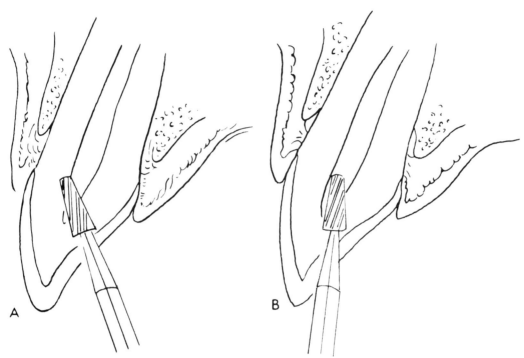

Figure 4–11 Possible approaches to the pulp chamber of the maxillary central incisor by gaining access through the lingual surface.

A, The approach often attempted by centering the drill at a right angle to the lingual surface of the crown, with the intention of penetrating the incisal portion of the pulp chamber. This is an improper approach to the problem. Since the pulp chamber is narrow at that point, it will almost invariably be bypassed, with a false step created in the labial surface of the pulp chamber. Because the ultimate opening must be in line with the pulp chamber and canal in order to allow the proper insertion of canal instruments, the alignment of the initial penetration must be compatible with that plan.

B, This picture shows the proper approach to the pulp chamber and the relationship of drill and linguoincisal surface in order to open the pulp cavity as nearly in line with the root canal as possible. The drill is to be held parallel to the crown and root axis, starting the penetration immediately lingual to the incisal ridge, the aim being to enter the cavity above the pulp chamber roof. Any remaining undercut of the roof portion can be smoothed out and cleaned after proper access has been created to involve the major portion of the pulp cavity (Figs. 4–12 and 4–13).

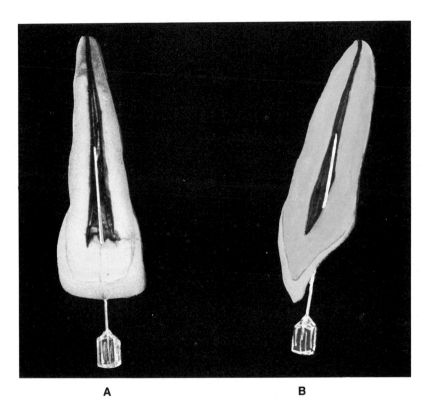

A   **B**

Figure 4–12 Maxillary central incisor—two aspects with simulated root canal instruments inserted into the pulp cavities.

A, Mesiodistal cross section of actual specimen. A simulated root canal instrument is shown placed into the cavity parallel with the long axis of the tooth viewed from the labial aspect.

B, A drawing portraying a labiolingual cross section of a maxillary central incisor with a simulated canal instrument in the relationship it would take when placed through the lingual opening as suggested in Figure 4–11, *B.* Note the variation in pulp cavity design by comparing *A* and *B.*

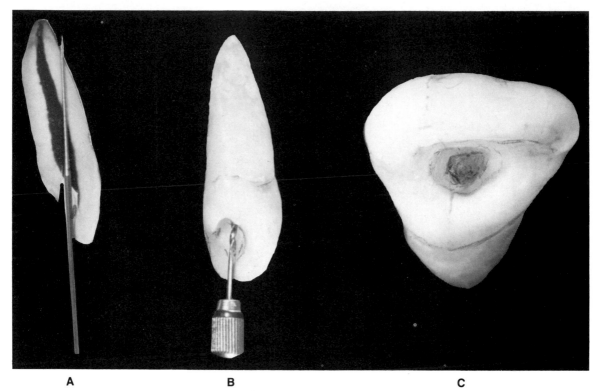

A   **B**   **C**

Figure 4–13 Instrument approach to the pulp cavity of the maxillary central incisor.

A, Photo of a labiolingual section of a maxillary central incisor. A straight probe is placed over a simulated lingual opening to show the need for instrument flexibility in order to follow the pulp canal path.

B, A root canal reamer is placed in a natural central incisor with the liberal lingual opening as suggested. Even with the generous opening, the instrument fits tightly against the linguoincisal portion of the crown in its attempt to follow the root canal.

C, An enlarged photo of a natural maxillary central incisor, incisal aspect. Proper entry has been made in line with the pulp chamber and root canal. The operator administering endodontic treatment must realize, however, that curvature exists beyond view. Check this aspect with *A* and *B*.

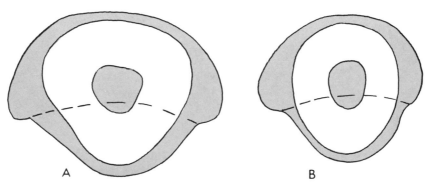

A   **B**

Figure 4–14 *See opposite page for legend.*

1   2   3   4   5

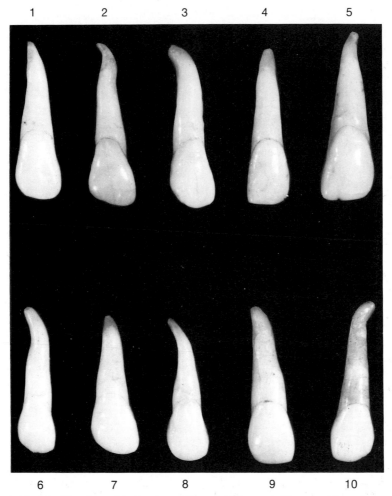

6   7   8   9   10

Figure 4–15 Maxillary lateral incisor—root form, labial aspect. Here are 10 good examples of the typical root form and development of the maxillary lateral incisor. The roots are slender when viewed from the labial aspect because they are extensions of the limited mesiodistal calibrations of the crown forms. The roots taper evenly for about two-thirds of their length, whereupon they taper more rapidly, forming a pointed tip apically. In most of these teeth this pointed tip will curve somewhat, usually in a distal direction (2, 10). Some tips are quite straight from the labial aspect (1, 4, 7).

Figure 4–14 A comparison of tooth form proportions in the maxillary central and lateral incisors.
A, Maxillary central incisor, incisal aspect.
B, Maxillary lateral incisor, incisal aspect.
The overall proportions of each tooth crown are shown in silhouette as they might be in a mirrored view looking incisally in line with the long axis of the teeth. The outlines of cervical portions of such teeth are superimposed in white over the shaded crowns in the relationship they would assume to the crown dimensions. Root canals are also shaded and centered in the proper relationship to incisal ridges. Note also the variation in size and shape of the central incisor cervical portion versus that of the lateral incisor.

1   2   3   4   5

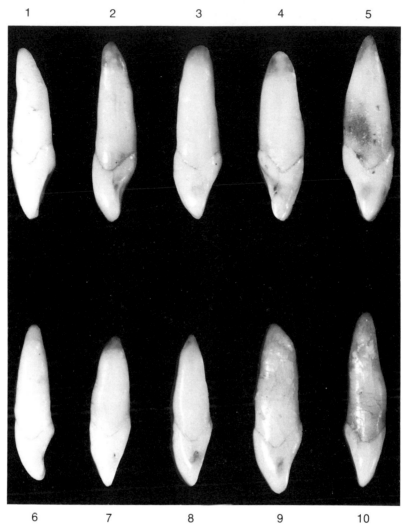

6   7   8   9   10

Figure 4–16 Maxillary lateral incisor—root form, mesial aspect. The labiolingual calibration of maxillary lateral incisor roots is quite generous, conforming to all the other anterior teeth in design. The broad crowns and roots, when viewed from the mesial aspect, reinforce and strengthen the units against forces brought to bear against them in a faciolingual direction. The tapering of the root from this aspect is very gradual, the labial and lingual sides being almost parallel at times. The root tips look rather blunt from the mesial or distal aspect. Some of these lateral roots will bend labially at the apical third (see 1 and 2). This formation is not apparent in radiographs taken in the usual manner.

Figure 4–18 Maxillary lateral incisor, cross sections of natural specimens.
A, 1 to 6, Labiolingual sections. This aspect does not show in radiographs taken the standard way.
B, 1 to 6, Mesiodistal sections.
C, 1 to 6, Cervical sections of root.
D, 1 to 6, Midroot sections.

Figure 4-17 Maxillary lateral incisor, labial aspect and distal aspect.

Normal pulp cavity forms are painted on the tooth surfaces as they might be seen normally in the cross sections. Note the comparison between the spacing and the form of the pulp chamber portion in the crown of one aspect as distinguished from the other. The labial or lingual aspect shows the pulp chamber portion to be wide, reflecting the crown outline. Viewed from the mesial or distal aspect, in a comparison of the crown and root portions of the pulp cavity, the cervical third portion of the root canal is wider than the same portion viewed from the labial or lingual in a mesiodistal cross section. The pulp chamber portion is narrow and pointed toward the incisal ridge.

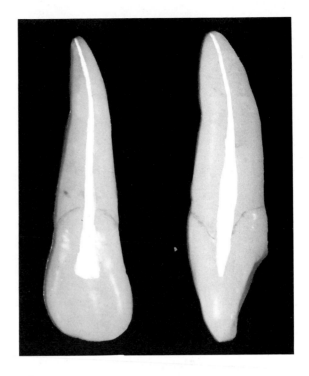

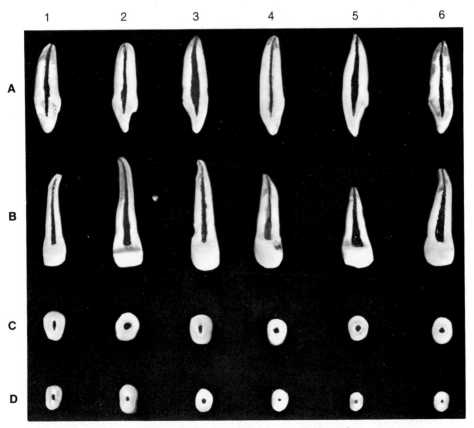

Figure 4-18 *See opposite page for legend.*

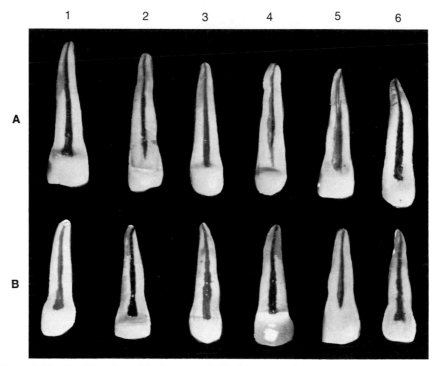

Figure 4–19   Maxillary lateral incisors, mesiodistal cross sections.

Because of their similarity in function, the pulp cavities of maxillary lateral incisors and maxillary central incisors bear a close resemblance to each other. Therefore, the general form of the pulp cavities will reflect that similarity. Dimensionally the lateral incisor is smaller than the central except for its root length. The lateral incisor root is always the more slender, but longer accordingly than that of the central incisor; the root length of the average central incisor is approximately one and one-third that of the crown, whereas the lateral incisor root can be one and one-half to nearly twice the length of its crown portion.

Because the root is narrow, the root canal as displayed by the mesiodistal section will be rather slender, but as a rule it will allow the penetration of instruments, no constriction interfering under normal conditions (Note exception in *A, 4*). There is one distinction when comparing this aspect to that of the central incisor: the pulp chamber of the lateral incisor will usually show a rounded form incisally, seldom showing evidences of a form to accommodate pulp horns.

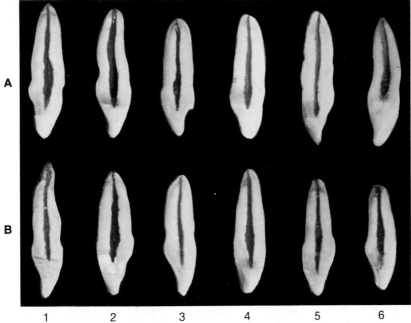

Figure 4–20 Maxillary lateral incisor, labiolingual cross sections. Comparison with the maxillary central incisor from this aspect may be made by observing Figure 4–7. The size of the pulp cavities will vary from that of the maxillary central incisors in direct ratio to crown and root measurements. The general shape of the spaces for pulp accommodations are quite similar.

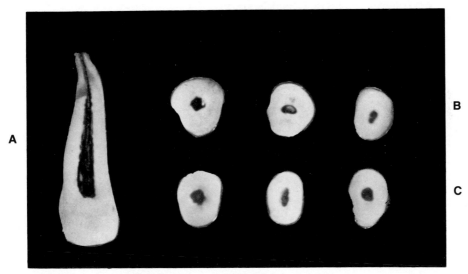

Figure 4–21 Maxillary lateral incisor, cross sections.

A, Mesiodistal cross section of a natural tooth specimen showing a pulp cavity of generous proportions. Note the definite rounded form of the pulp chamber portion which shows no definite pulp horn development. There is no demarcation between the pulp chamber and the pulp canal; this formation is typical of single-rooted teeth.

B and *C,* Six cervical cross sections made at the juncture of crown and root. Some will resemble small maxillary central incisors, others small maxillary canines. The lateral incisor seems to be vestigial in character; at times, even the crown will vary in form; in one instance, it will resemble a dwarf central incisor; at another time, it will resemble a small maxillary canine.

Although crown forms of the maxillary lateral incisor will vary considerably in formation, usually the roots are smoothly formed and of good length.

87

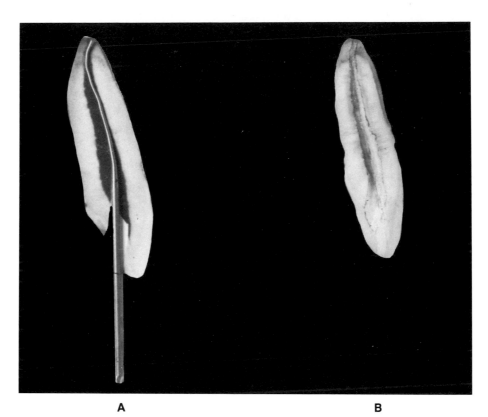

A   **B**

Figure 4–22   Maxillary lateral incisor, two views.

A, Photo of a labiolingual section of a maxillary lateral incisor. A smooth broach is placed to simulate entrance through a lingual opening in the tooth crown, showing the bending of the broach required in order to follow the pulp cavity to its apical terminal. Compare this with Figure 4–13, *A.*

B, Photo of another natural maxillary lateral incisor which has been dissected. The labiolingual section exposes the pulp cavity, including the directional approach lingually required to accomplish proper entry of canal instruments. Note the similarity between *A* and *B.*

CHAPTER 5

Maxillary Premolars

The two maxillary premolars bear a close relationship in their anatomical characteristics. The pulp cavity design reflects this similarity, even though detailed descriptions of the design as shown by cross sections of the two are not identical. Each of the maxillary premolars can be characterized so that certain probabilities can be anticipated in the endodontic diagnosis of the cavity form.

These maxillary teeth must be placed high on the list of possible casualties with pulp involvement. Although protected somewhat from extraneous injury by the guardianship of the powerful canines, they may be subject to other problems. They are "caries-prone" for one thing. Their crown forms display areas that often allow carious inroads, broad interproximal spaces, and deep developmental grooves. Because the maxillary first premolar has long cusps divided by the deep developmental occlusal grooves, and accented developmental depressions mesially separating the buccal and lingual root portions, this tooth is subject to fracture. Often the injury is autogenous, taking place during normal mastication. Naturally, if the crown is weakened by caries or restoration procedures, breakage of one type or another is even more likely.

Then, too, the maxillary premolars can be valuable as dental appliance abutments. The abutments can be made more useful sometimes if dowels or pins are utilized, preceded by endodontic preparation.

The calcification and development of the maxillary first and second premolars are presented in Figure 5–1 and in the tables on this page and page 91.

MAXILLARY FIRST PREMOLAR

CALCIFICATION OF MAXILLARY FIRST PREMOLAR

First evidence of calcification	1½ to 1¾ years
Enamel completed	5 to 6 years
Eruption	10 to 11 years
Root completed	12 to 13 years

CROSS-SECTIONAL ANATOMY: DESIGN OF PULP CAVITIES (Fig. 5–6, *A, B, C, D, E*)

Buccolingual Cross Section (Fig. 5–6, *A, D*)

The maxillary first premolar may have two well-developed and fully formed roots, one buccal and one lingual. Most often, there will be two root projections apically from the middle third of the root portion. Although it is not uncommon for this tooth to possess one broad root for its entire length, rarely does it have less than two separated root canals for the major portion of the root length (Fig. 5–6, *A,* 4, 6). This cross section will display a broad pulp chamber buccolingually with accommodations for well-developed pulp horns in the roof of the chamber. Only when secondary deposit is extensive will this form be absent. Teeth with the most distinct separate root development will have relatively shallow pulp chambers (Fig. 5–6, *A,* 2, 9). Characteristically, all root canals in this tooth, regardless of root form, will have smooth, funnel-like openings leading into the canals from the pulp chamber floor.

A comparison of pulp chambers in this tooth is interesting. The teeth with the least root separation will usually have the deepest pulp chambers (Fig. 5–6, *A,* 4; *D,* 18). The age of the patient and the comparison of root length must also be considered in these cases.

The pulp chamber floor will be below the level of the cementoenamel junction where cervical cross sections are made. This design puts the floor considerably below the normal gum line in vivo.

The root canals taper evenly from the floor of the pulp chamber to the end of the root form. The lingual root canal tends to be larger, regardless of the root form. The teeth with the least root spread will have the straightest pulp canals, with a tendency toward parallelism in those that are fused more completely (Fig. 5–7, *A,* 3, 4).

Mesiodistal Cross Section (Fig. 5–6, *B, E*)

The shape of the pulp cavity of the maxillary first premolar, when viewing a mesiodistal cross section, shows a cavity similar to the maxillary canine; it is relatively narrow with an even taper from pulp chamber to root end. Since the root is shorter and since the overall measurement is less than that of the canine, the pulp cavity will vary accordingly.

Pulp stones and secondary dentin deposit may cause difficulty in the endodontic procedure (Fig. 5–6, *B,* 4, 8; *E,* 14, 17).

Cervical Cross Section (Fig. 5–6, C)

The cross section at the cervical line made transversely through the root at the cementoenamel junction demonstrates the outline form of the root trunk as it joins the crown of the tooth. The maxillary first premolar has a characteristic root outline at this level. Usually it is kidney-shaped. This form is assisted by a deep indentation mesially that is part of a developmental depression which extends upward into the cervical third of the crown mesially, above the cervical cut (Fig. 5–8, 3). The root form cervically is wider buccolingually than mesiodistally with a constricted crescent-shaped pulp chamber centered in it (Fig. 5–10, 2).

MAXILLARY SECOND PREMOLAR

CALCIFICATION OF THE MAXILLARY SECOND PREMOLAR

First evidence of calcification	2 to 2¼ years
Enamel completed	6 to 7 years
Eruption	10 to 12 years
Root completed	12 to 14 years

CROSS-SECTIONAL ANATOMY: DESIGN OF PULP CAVITIES (Fig. 5–16, A, B, C, D, E)

Buccolingual Cross Section (Fig. 5–16, A, D)

A comparison of maxillary premolar pulp cavities in buccolingual cross section brings out some interesting points. The two maxillary premolars are not alike. They cannot be compared in the same manner, as can the mandibular central and lateral incisors. It is rare to find bifurcated roots in this tooth, although it is not uncommon to find two pulp canals, one buccal and one lingual. This aspect shows one feature common to the first premolars, and that is the shape of the roof of the pulp chamber, which accommodates two well-developed pulp horns, one for each cusp, buccal and lingual. The rest of the pulp cavity of the second premolar is not comparable. From this aspect, the average pulp cavity is very broad at its junction with the pulp chamber, and then it narrows very gradually, remaining quite wide until it reaches midroot or beyond. There it constricts rapidly, becoming a typical root canal in diameter as it approaches the apical third of the root (see Fig. 5–16, A, 1, 6, 8). In most cases, the canal is approachable apically; sometimes the apical foramen itself seems quite open. This possibility should be kept in mind in order to avoid unnecessary tissue trauma. This is a departure from a similar situation in the maxillary first premolar (see Fig. 5–16, *A*, 2, 7; *D*, 12, 17, 18). Sometimes the pulp canal of the second premolar branches into accessory canals near the apical end (Fig. 5–16, *D*, 10, 15, 16). Endodontists will be interested in another characteristic found in the maxillary second premolars when a study is made of their pulp cavities and root formations. Buccolingual cross sections will be found with the single broad pulp canal divided at midroot into two canals by a dentin "island" (Fig. 5–16, *A*, 5; *D*, 15, 17). Then, moving apically, the two canals join again and become one as the apical third of the root is approached. This explains why at times a root canal instrument working through the crown of the tooth may seem to penetrate one time and then seems obstructed the next. Deliberate manipulation will coax the instrument to bypass the obstruction. The buccolingual cross section is produced by cutting half the tooth away; therefore, what appears as an "island" is actually a bar of dentin connecting the two halves in situ. An instrument must bypass the bar on both the buccal and lingual sides.

Mesiodistal Cross Section (Fig. 5–16, *B*, *E*)

There seems to be no variation in the appearance of the pulp cavity in the mesiodistal section of the second maxillary premolar as distinguished from the maxillary first premolar. The cavity appears slender, becoming even narrower as it approaches the root end. Any difficulty encountered in penetrating root canals in this tooth because of constriction can usually be attributed to the known form of the canals as seen from this aspect in the dental radiograph (Fig. 5–16, *B*, 2, 7; *E*, 11, 12, 15).

Cervical Cross Section (Fig. 5–16, *C*)

The cervical cross section of the maxillary second premolar generally will demonstrate a root trunk that is smoothly oval in shape (Fig. 5–16, *C*, 2, 4, 7). A few will show a crimp in the mesial or distal side of the root, but none will approach the kidney shape of the maxillary first premolar (Fig. 5–16, *C*, 1, 3). The pulp chamber will be centered in the root, and the shape will correlate with the outline of the root but in miniature.

SUMMARY – MAXILLARY PREMOLARS

The maxillary premolars bear a close relationship in their anatomical characteristics. The pulp cavity design reflects this similarity, even though detailed descriptions of the design as shown by cross sections of the two are not identical. Each of the maxillary premolars can be characterized so that in endodontic diagnosis certain probabilities of the cavity form can be anticipated.

Maxillary premolars often require endodontic treatment. The first premolar is subject to fracture because of its formation. The long sharp cusps are divided by a deep occlusal sulcus and developmental groove. This form is further complicated by a developmental groove in the mesial marginal ridge and a deep developmental depression mesially that is often a continuation of a root bifurcation. The "lines of cleavage" thus produced foster the possibility of fracture from any force applied sharply in a buccolingual direction.

Maxillary premolars can be valuable as dental appliance abutments. At times patient requirements may suggest endodontic interference. Fundamentally, the pulp cavities of both teeth will bear a resemblance; for instance, the overall form of the cavities will be broad buccolingually and narrow mesiodistally. Nevertheless, in nearly every case, the maxillary first premolar will exhibit two root canals, whereas the second premolar will usually show only one, at least for most of its root length (Fig. 5–16, *A, D*).

The approach to the pulp cavities in the maxillary premolars is not difficult. Root canal instruments can be applied in line with the straight root forms. Any interference encountered would be due to the branching of root canals or to blockage caused by the secondary deposit of dentin.

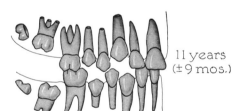

11 years
(±9 mos.)

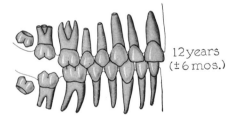

12 years
(±6 mos.)

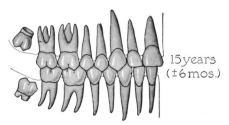

15 years
(±6 mos.)

Figure 5–1 The calcification and development of maxillary first and second premolars. This portion of the Schour and Massler chart shows, among other things, the development of the roots of maxillary premolars from the ages of 11 to 15 years. Until the apical ends of roots are mature, there is always some risk associated with endodontic treatment. (From The development of human dentition. J.A.D.A., *28*:1153–1160, 1941, by I. Shour and M. Massler, University of Illinois College of Dentistry.)

MAXILLARY FIRST PREMOLARS

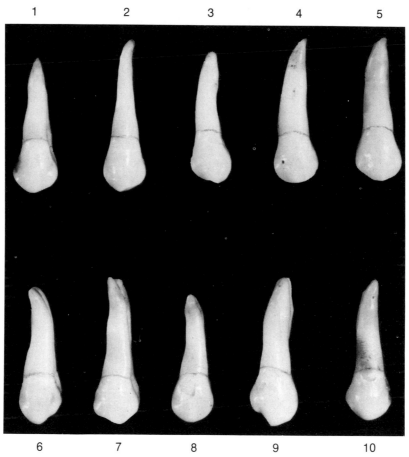

Figure 5–2 Maxillary first premolars—root forms of 10 typical specimens, buccal aspect.
From this aspect, the roots taper rather evenly, usually bending distally at the apical third. Most have roots of good length, approximately one and one-half times the crown length from cervical line to cusp tip. The first premolar roots from this aspect look single and slender, which, of course, is not a true picture. Dental radiographs can promote the same impression. Figure 5–3 shows these specimens viewed from the mesial aspect.

1   2   3   4   5

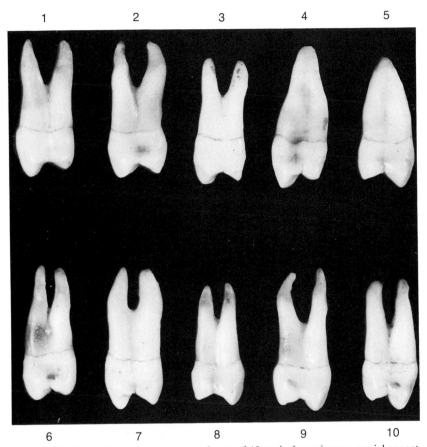

6   7   8   9   10

Figure 5–3 Maxillary first premolars — root forms of 10 typical specimens, mesial aspect.
    Although they are not lined up in exactly the same manner, these are the same teeth shown in Figure 5–2. From this aspect the root form differs entirely from the impression given by the buccal aspect. There seem to be three distinct types of root form: well-separated roots, one buccal, and one lingual; one broad, single root for half or more of its length with the apical portion bifurcated; and one root which is broad buccolingually, ending in a bluntly tapered apical end. The last type is seen less often. Buccolingual cross sections show that all three types have two distinct root canals, regardless of the root form.

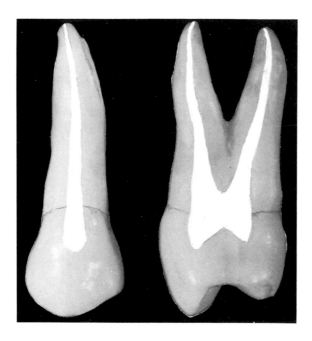

Figure 5–4 Maxillary first premolar, buccal aspect and mesial aspect. The typical pulp cavity form is painted on the surfaces of the tooth as it might appear in cross section from the two aspects. The contrast between the two views is quite noticeable. The standard technique for dental radiographs will not show the complicated pulp cavity form as depicted in a buccolingual cross section.

Figure 5–5 Maxillary first premolar. The shaded area represents the occlusal opening that is desirable for convenient access to the pulp cavity. If the tooth crown is intact, the opening will take in the developmental groove formation, stay just inside the marginal formations mesially and distally, and then include the transverse ridge of the occlusal surface up to the occlusal slopes of the two cusp tips. The area will approximate the outline advocated by Black for an occlusal restoration. This extension will not be required in order to properly enter the root canals with instruments (as was necessary for first molars). However, another problem of convenience enters the picture: the occlusal surface between cusps is minimal; therefore, the opening for access must be emphasized in order to mirror the field of operation centered in the pulp chamber. At times, in maxillary premolars the pulp chamber portion of the pulp cavity can be quite deep and difficult to handle in the operative procedure. *Because the crown forms of both maxillary premolars are similar in occlusal area, this illustration will suffice for each of them when discussing occlusal access for the approach to pulp cavities.*

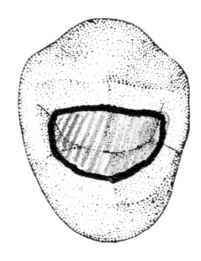

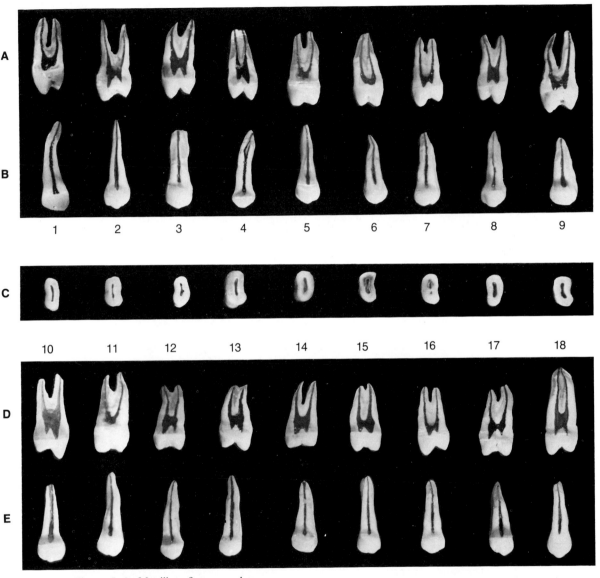

Figure 5–6 Maxillary first premolar.

A, Buccolingual cross section, exposing the mesial or distal aspect of the pulp cavity. This aspect does not show on standard dental radiographs.

B, Mesiodistal cross section, exposing the buccal or lingual aspect of the pulp cavity.

C, Cervical cross section. A transverse cut at the cementoenamel junction exposing the pulp chamber. These are the openings to root canals that will be seen in the floor of the pulp chamber.

D, Buccolingual cross section, exposing the mesial or distal aspect of the pulp cavity.

E, Mesiodistal cross section, exposing the buccal or lingual aspect of the pulp cavity.

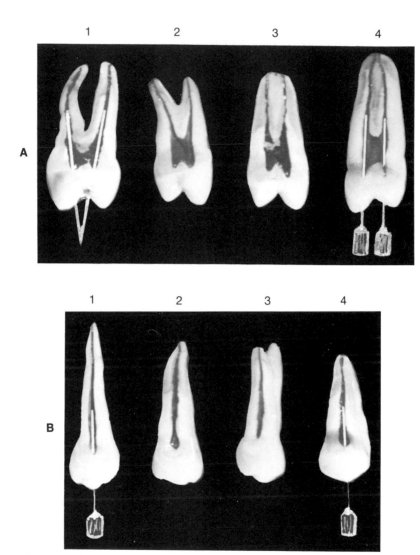

Figure 5–7 Maxillary first premolar, buccolingual and mesiodistal cross sections.

  A, Four typical cross sections with cuts made buccolingually showing probable pulp cavity form to be expected in each type. The first specimen with completely separated roots will require an angled approach with instruments. This type has a shallow pulp chamber. The second one has the most common form of root separation for this tooth. In this case the pulp chamber is deep and the greater part of the two root canals could be traversed in a parallel manner. The third and fourth specimens are the single-root type — one with two apical foramina and one with two nearly parallel canals coming together at the long root end. In the latter type, the two root canal instruments would be relatively parallel during full penetration.

  B, These four mesiodistal cross sections display similar typical pulp cavity forms. The narrow tapering forms from this aspect will follow a rather straight path from the pulp chamber to the root apex.

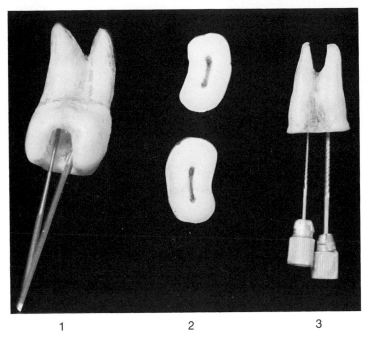

1   2   3

Figure 5–8 Maxillary first premolar.

1, Odd angle view of the maxillary first premolar, showing the approach to the root canals with instruments placed within a generous opening made in the occlusal surface of the crown. Some bifurcation of the roots with two distinct canals is characteristic of this tooth.

2, Cervical sections of two of these teeth, one right and one left. At this point the root form is noticeably kidney-shaped, with the mesial surface curved in toward the pulp chamber. This developmental depression, reflected also in the cervical third of the mesial surface of the crown, is characteristic of this tooth alone (see Fig. 5–9).

3, Instruments are placed in the two canals with the crown cut away as an added demonstration. Note the depression showing cervically on the root.

Figure 5–9 Maxillary first premolar. Another view of two of the specimens shown in Figure 5–8. Sometimes a fresh view from a new perspective is desirable. A straight profile pose of the premolar accents the mesial surface of crown and root. One root canal instrument is deeply inserted in the buccal root.

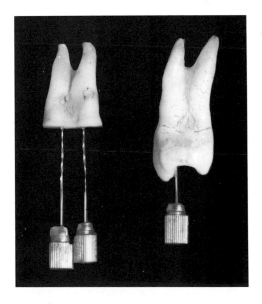

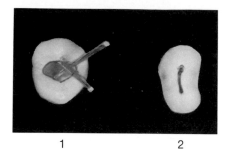

1   2

Figure 5–10 Maxillary first premolar.

1, Occlusal opening as advocated in a natural specimen. Instruments have been placed in root canals; the variation in the angle of approach is greater than usual. This approach is more likely if the pulp cavity is divided by an "island," or if the tooth has two well-separated roots (see Fig. 5–7, *A*, 1).

2, Typical cervical cross section.

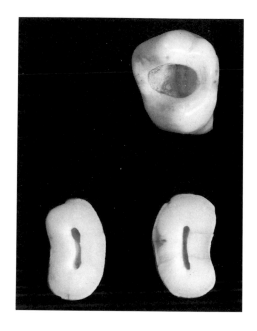

Figure 5–11 Maxillary first premolar. Three specimens are shown—one with the crown opened occlusally as if for endodontic treatment, and two cervical sections with crowns removed at the cementoenamel junction buccally and lingually. A clear picture of the pulp chamber through the large occlusal opening is very difficult to obtain. This furnishes a good reason for the advocacy of cavity extension in order to facilitate endodontic treatment. The operator needs all the help available in order to properly mirror the view and to apply instrumentation (Figs. 5–8 and 5–10).

The two cervical sections, one a right first premolar and one a left, display clearly the crescent shape of the pulp cavity that is typical for this tooth at the cervical level.

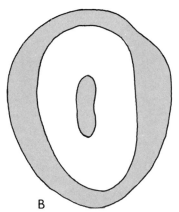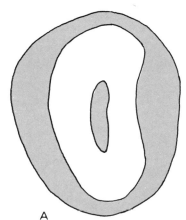

B   A

Figure 5–12 A comparison of tooth form proportions in the maxillary premolars.

A, Maxillary first premolar, occlusal aspect.

B, Maxillary second premolar, occlusal aspect.

The overall proportions of each tooth crown are shown in silhouette as they might be seen in a mirrored view looking occlusally in line with long axes of the teeth. The outline of cervical portions of each tooth are superimposed in white over the shaded crowns in a dimensional relationship. Pulp chamber openings are shaded also and placed in proper relation to occlusal surfaces. Note the variation in cervical form between the two premolars. The first premolar assumes a kidney shape with a major indentation mesially (see Fig. 5–8).

100

MAXILLARY SECOND PREMOLARS

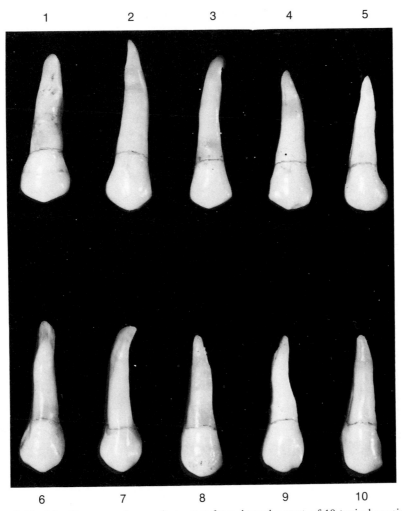

Figure 5–13 Maxillary second premolars—root form, buccal aspect, of 10 typical specimens.
From this aspect the roots, like those of the first premolar, taper rather evenly, tending to bend distally at the apical third. Most of these roots are of good length, often exceeding those of the maxillary first premolars. The roots of these specimens appear quite different from the mesial aspect shown in Figure 5–14.

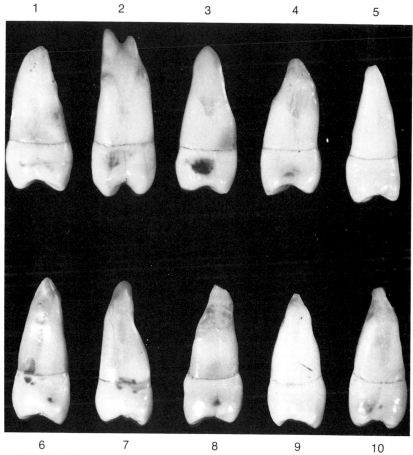

Figure 5–14 Maxillary second premolars—root form, mesial aspect, of 10 typical specimens.
From this aspect the root form differs entirely from the impression given of these teeth in Figure 5–13. Usually the root appears broad and single with a gradual taper, ending in a bluntly pointed apical end. Only occasionally will there be a hint of bifurcation at the root tip (2). This type would have two apical foramina, differing from most maxillary second premolars with one foramen.

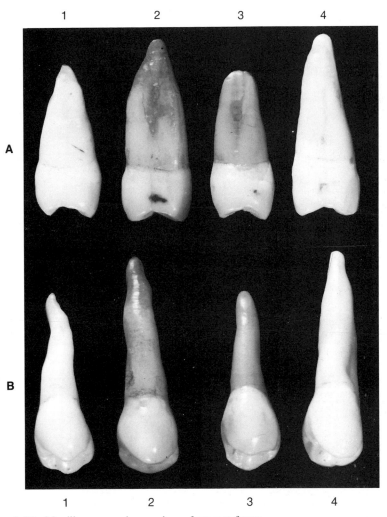

Figure 5–15 Maxillary second premolars—four root forms.

A, Mesial aspect.

1, Relatively short root, tapers rapidly from the crown cervix to a pointed apical end. Pointed root tips usually indicate a single apical foramen.

2, Relatively long root having nearly parallel buccal and lingual sides for about half its length before tapering rapidly to a pointed apex.

3, Relatively short root with a gradual taper buccally and lingually, ending in a very blunt apex. This type usually has divided root canals and duplicate foramina.

4, A very long root. The description of specimen 1, in regard to root form and pulp cavity form, would be applicable to this specimen as well.

B, Lingual aspect.

1, Root displays considerable curvature.

2, The root shows a resemblance from this aspect to its design as described from the mesial aspect; the sides of the root remain nearly parallel until a rapid tapering takes place in the upper half.

3, The root tapers very gradually, ending in a blunt apex; this design is consistent with that shown from the mesial aspect.

4, This long root has mesial and distal sides approaching parallelism for most of its length. This is not consistent with its design from the mesial aspect. Also, it has a developmental depression mesially not found usually on a maxillary second premolar.

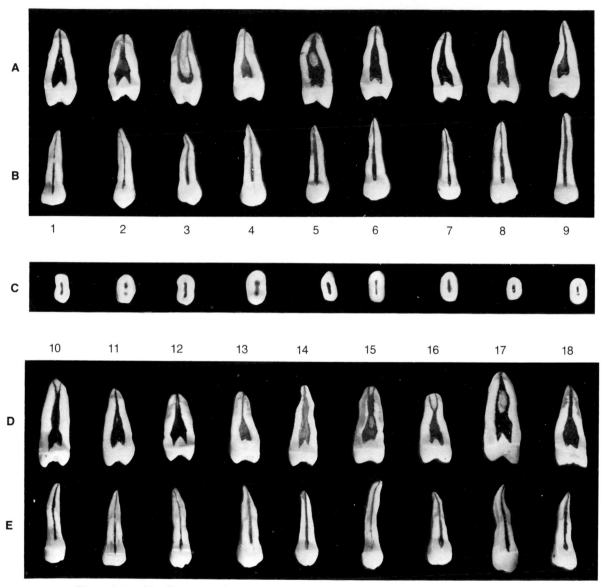

Figure 5–16 Maxillary second premolar.

A, Buccolingual cross section, exposing the mesial or distal aspect of the pulp cavity. This aspect does not show on standard dental radiographs.

B, Mesiodistal cross section, exposing the buccal or lingual aspect of the pulp cavity.

C, Cervical cross section. A transverse cut at the cementoenamel junction exposing the pulp chamber. These are the openings to root canals that will be seen in the floor of the pulp chamber.

D, Buccolingual cross section, exposing the mesial or distal aspect of the pulp cavity.

E, Mesiodistal cross section, exposing the buccal or lingual aspect of the pulp cavity.

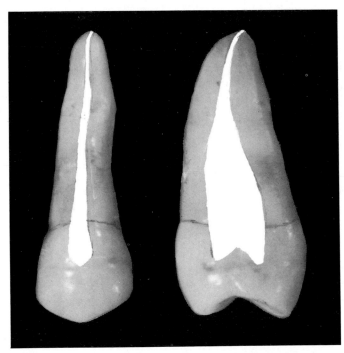

Figure 5–17 Maxillary second premolar, buccal aspect and mesial aspect. The typical pulp cavity form is painted on the tooth surfaces as they might appear in cross section from the two aspects. The contrast between the two views is quite noticeable. The buccolingual cross section shows a typical anatomical variation possessed by the maxillary second premolar. The pulp chamber portion shows no division into canals as it traverses the greater portion of the root. The cavity narrows rapidly near the apical third, tapering until it becomes a constricted apical portion with one foramen. This formation is not invariable, of course (Fig. 5–16, *A, D*).

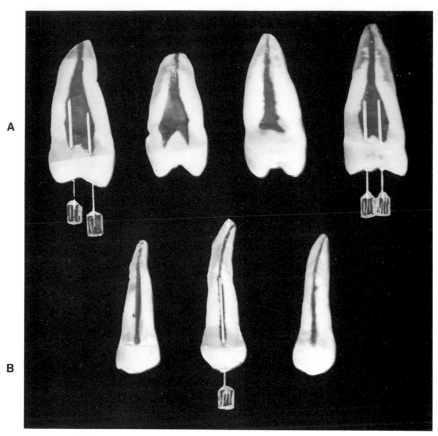

Figure 5-18 Maxillary second premolar, buccolingual and mesiodistal cross sections.

A, Four typical specimens with cuts made buccolingually showing the probable pulp cavity form to be found in the maxillary second premolar. The first specimen shows simulated root canal instruments penetrating about half the root length in the wide pulp cavity buccolingually. From that area, the instruments would have to bend in order to follow the constriction as the root canal tapers apically. The other specimens in *A* show some variance in the cavity outlines, but fundamentally they are similar (Fig. 5-16, *A*, *D*). These specimens demonstrate very well the tendency of apical foramina to show visible width buccolingually in second premolars.

B, Three typical specimens with cuts made mesiodistally displaying typical pulp cavity forms. The center tooth with a long root is curved a little more than average, starting at midroot. However, the curvature is gradual and would present no problem if properly flexible instruments were used.

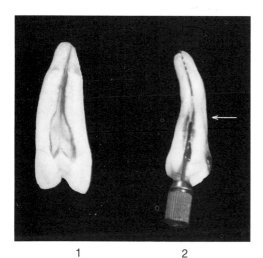

Figure 5-19 Maxillary second premolar, two interesting specimens.

1, Buccolingual section showing a typical formation of the pulp cavity; however, many of these teeth would have a greater extension of the wide portion toward the apex (Figs. 5-17 and 5-18).

2, A mesiodistal cross section with a root canal instrument in full penetration of the curved pulp cavity. The reamer has bypassed an "island," which is indicated by an arrow pointing toward it. Such a phenomenon is often encountered in teeth with broad roots similar to the maxillary second premolar (Fig. 5-16, *A*, 5; *D*, 15, 17).

106

Figure 5–20 Maxillary second premolar. Two views with root canal instruments.

1, The instruments remain parallel, with about one-half penetration of the root. The crown has been removed at the cementoenamel junction. Most of these teeth will have one broad canal buccolingually for some distance before it bifurcates or narrows to one slender canal (Fig. 5–16, *A*, *D*).

2, Here an instrument is inserted until perforation of the apical foramen is obtained. Note the alignment of the instrument shaft, with placement close to the lingual side of the occlusal opening. A typical characteristic of the pulp cavity of the maxillary second premolar should also be noted: the lingual wall of the cavity assumes a line almost straight with the apical constriction, whereas the buccal wall extends buccally and curves considerably before traveling in a lingual direction to join the apical constriction (Fig. 5–19, 1, and several specimens in Fig. 5–16, *A*, *D*).

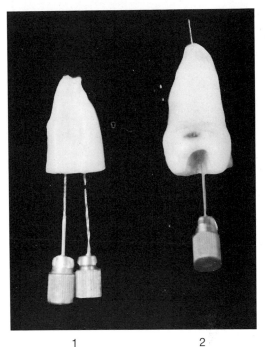

1   2

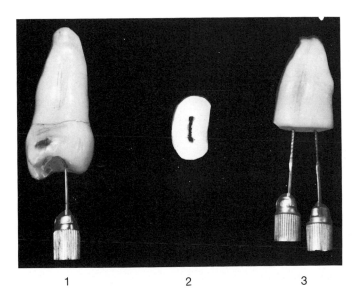

1   2   3

Figure 5–21 Maxillary second premolar.

1, Position of instrument as it enters single broad canal through a comparatively wide occlusal opening buccolingually. Notice how the instrument hugs the lingual side. Sometimes the broad canal buccolingually will branch as it progresses apically.

2, Cross section of root at cementoenamel junction. It is slightly kidney-shaped with elongated pulp chamber, but it is less extreme in this respect than the maxillary first premolar.

3, Two root canal instruments placed partially parallel in the broad canal with the crown removed for clarity of observation.

CHAPTER 6

Mandibular Premolars

Although they share the same functional area in the mandible, the first and second premolars differ somewhat in functional form.

The first premolar usually has a root of modest length, somewhat round on cross section, which could make the tooth unstable if counter forces were applied to it. However, occlusal forces against this tooth are limited by its crown form. The main occlusal contact is limited by the pointed buccal cusp; the small lingual cusp being nonfunctional.

The mandibular first premolar is a candidate for endodontic treatment on occasion. Two possibilities for pulp involvement can be mentioned. Caries can make inroads in vulnerable interproximal areas and in the developmental grooves on the linguo-occlusal surface. Morphologically, the pulp horn responsible for the tall cusp formation is, at times, so near that surface that very little penetration is necessary from caries or by dental bur in order to accomplish pulp involvement. In fact, accidental injury to the pulp by dental bur is a frequent cause of pulp involvement encountered in mandibular first premolars. For instance, a relatively shallow cut made into the developmental occlusal grooves for caries removal or for a filling anchorage can be a dangerous approach toward the prominent buccal pulp horn. Exposure is easily acquired (Fig. 6–6).

The mandibular first premolar can present another endodontic problem, based on probabilities in development. Branching root canals and even root bifurcations are not uncommon. These variations in root form are difficult to diagnose from standard dental radiographs (Figs. 6–9 and 6–10).

The mandibular second premolar is a larger, stronger tooth than the first premolar, having a thick bulky crown with a completely functional occlusal surface. Its root is strongly built for anchorage, and it is as long or longer than the root of any other posterior tooth in the mandible (Fig. 6–12).

Because this tooth is a strong functioning unit as part of the

108

occlusal mechanism, it is very useful, and consequently it is highly regarded by its host. Therefore, on occasion, conservation of the valuable mandibular second premolar will depend upon successful endodontic treatment.

MANDIBULAR FIRST PREMOLAR

CALCIFICATION OF THE MAXILLARY FIRST PREMOLAR

First evidence of calcification	1¾ to 2 years
Enamel completed	5 to 6 years
Eruption	10 to 12 years
Root completed	12 to 13 years

CROSS-SECTIONAL ANATOMY: DESIGN OF PULP CAVITIES (Fig. 6–4, *A, B, C, D, E*)

Buccolingual Cross Section (Fig. 6–4, *A, D*)

The mandibular first premolar looks like a small mandibular canine with a dwarfed lingual cusp that is nonfunctional. Therefore, one would expect to find a pulp cavity which might be comparable to that of the canine. This is the situation, except for the smaller dimensions of the pulp cavity in the premolar tooth. The buccolingual cross section of the mandibular first premolar has a pointed pulp chamber portion to accommodate a generous pulp horn which points toward the tip of the large, well-formed buccal cusp of the crown. A pulp horn formation associated with the small lingual cusp will be insignificant if present (Fig. 6–4, *A*, 7, 8).

As in the canine, this section indicates a broad root canal, showing the width of the pulp chamber, tapering as it progresses apically. The average premolar pulp canal will show constriction at about the halfway point of the rooth length (Fig. 6–5, mesial aspect). Some mandibular first premolars, like the mandibular canine, will have pulp canals that are quite broad buccolingually until the final approach to the apical end of the root (Fig. 6–4, *D*, 12, 14, 16). Occasionally the root form shows a tendency toward bifurcation or a broadening effect apically. The root canal may divide in these cases with dual foramina (Fig. 6–4, *A*, 9; *D*, 18) (see also Fig. 6–10).

Mesiodistal Cross Section (Fig. 6–4, *B, E*)

The mesiodistal cross section of the mandibular first premolar displays the typical form of pulp cavity seen in this section of all premolars. The pulp chamber and canal are narrower from this angle, tapering evenly until a constricted apical foramen is reached. The pulp canal usually affords easy penetration in endodontic treatment. If there is difficulty, it will most likely be caused by a constriction in this mesiodistal direction (Fig. 6–4, *B*, 5; *E*, 11, 14).

Cervical Cross Section (Fig. 6–4, *C*)

All premolars may vary in crown size in different persons. The larger teeth will usually have crowns and roots that are in proportion. The mandibular first premolar may appear small when compared to other teeth in the same mouth. The cervical cross sections of this tooth will show size variations when teeth from different persons are compared (Fig. 6–4, *C*, 3, 8). The overall design of the root from this angle will be that of a small mandibular canine, wider facially than lingually. The pulp canal is, of course, usually wider buccolingually than mesiodistally.

MANDIBULAR SECOND PREMOLARS

CALCIFICATION OF THE MANDIBULAR SECOND PREMOLAR

First evidence of calcification	2¼ to 2½ years
Enamel completed	6 to 7 years
Eruption	11 to 12 years
Root completed	13 to 14 years

CROSS-SECTIONAL ANATOMY: DESIGN OF PULP CAVITIES (Fig. 6–13, *A, B, C, D, E*)

Buccolingual Cross Section (Fig. 6–13, *A, D*)

In line with the added size of crown and root, the buccolingual cross section of the mandibular second premolar will reflect the added size when comparison is made with the pulp cavity of the mandibular first premolar. Except for this differentiation, a description of the second premolar pulp cavity will come close to being a repetition of the description of the pulp cavity of the mandibular first premolar. Two details that differ when viewing the buccolingual cross section can be noted: (1) from this angle the pulp chamber and wide canal are confined in most cases to the crown and upper part of the root, and (2) there is a tendency for the wide pulp canal to form a narrow path on the way to the root apex (Fig. 6–13, *A*, 1, 7). Some, of course, do not conform to this plan. Another anatomical detail differs in a second premolar as distinguished from a first mandibular premolar: the roofs of the pulp chambers are pointed to accommodate more than one pulp horn in most cases (Fig. 6–13, *D*, 10, 13). This design coincides with the generous cusp development buccally and lingually in the second mandibular premolar. It is especially noticeable when making comparisons of lingual cusps of the two premolars.

Mesiodistal Cross Sections (Fig. 6–13, *B*, *E*)

Except for added root size and length and the obvious effect they would have on pulp cavity measurements, the description of the mesiodistal cross section of the mandibular second premolar is identical to that of the mandibular first premolar (and the mandibular canine). The root is often quite long and curved at the apical third. Although it may curve mesially or distally, it favors a distal direction.

Cervical Cross Section (Fig. 6–13, *C*)

The substantial root base in mandibular second premolars is, of course, reflected in the cross sections at the cementoenamel junction. Many of these specimens will resemble those of the mandibular canine even in overall dimensions. The calibrations are greater buccolingually than mesiodistally. The shape of the pulp chambers and root canals of these teeth resembles the outline of the root, but in miniature. Most of these root cross sections are consistently oval in character (in Fig. 6–18, compare *A*, 4, with *B*, 3).

SUMMARY – MANDIBULAR PREMOLARS

The mandibular first and second premolars are dissimilar.

The first premolar has a root of modest length with a single root canal, unless (which happens sometimes) the root is anomalous even to the point of bifurcation.

The strong buccal cusp of the mandibular first premolar houses a large pulp horn that could suffer from accidental exposure if the tooth were to be handled carelessly by the dental operator. The pulp cavity is quite narrow mesiodistally but of generous width buccolingually.

The mandibular second premolar is larger and stronger than the first premolar. Unlike the first, it has a completely functional occlusal surface, and the crown is supported by a root of considerable length and breadth. The pulp cavity centered in the larger tooth has proportionate development that adapts well to endodontic manipulation. The mandibular second premolar is very valuable as a contributor to dental maintenance and therefore is a good candidate for conservative treatment.

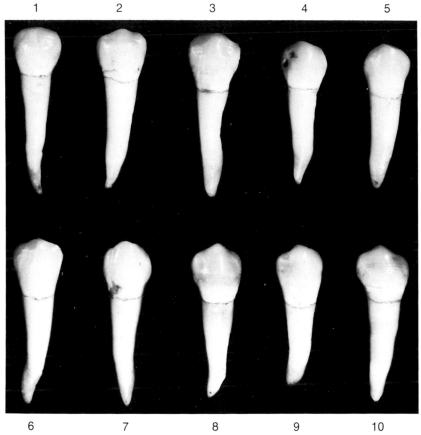

Figure 6–1   Mandibular first premolar—root form, buccal aspect. The root form of this tooth from the buccal aspect is tapered uniformly with the crown from the cementoenamel junction for most of its length. Near the apical third the root tip tapers more rapidly, ending in a comparatively sharp point. This latter portion exhibits some curvature, usually distal. The root length is sufficient for good anchorage, appearing quite long at times for a tooth of modest size.

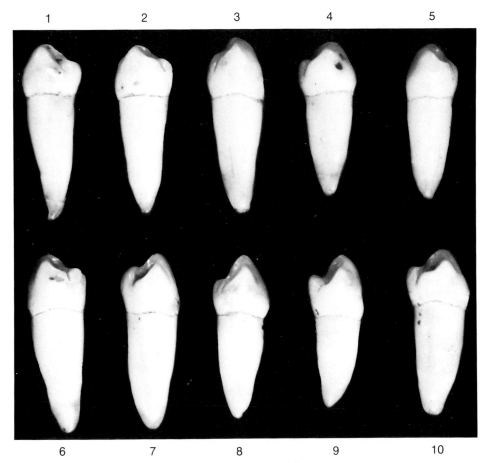

Figure 6–2 Mandibular first premolar—root form, mesial aspect.

From this aspect, the roots appear to have more generous proportions. Although the root of this tooth tapers evenly from the crown to the apex, it has more bulk buccolingually. The root tip may have either of two designs; it will exhibit a pointed or a rather blunt apex.

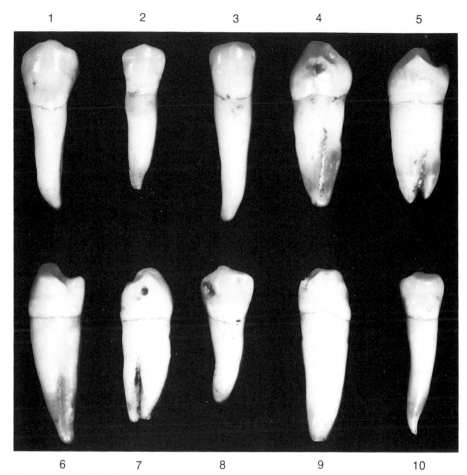

Figure 6–3 Mandibular first premolar—some variations of root form.

1, Root short for oversize crown.

2, Crown and root diminutive.

3, Root quite thick at cervix as it joins a flat-sided crown; root quite long also.

4, This root has a deep developmental groove mesially, which might indicate pulp canal complications.

5, Root with an actual bifurcation.

6, Root of extra length, deep developmental groove toward its end.

7, Root of average length but bifurcated.

8, Dwarfed root on full-sized crown.

9, Unusually long, powerful root for a first premolar.

10, A very long, curved root with a sharp, curved tip.

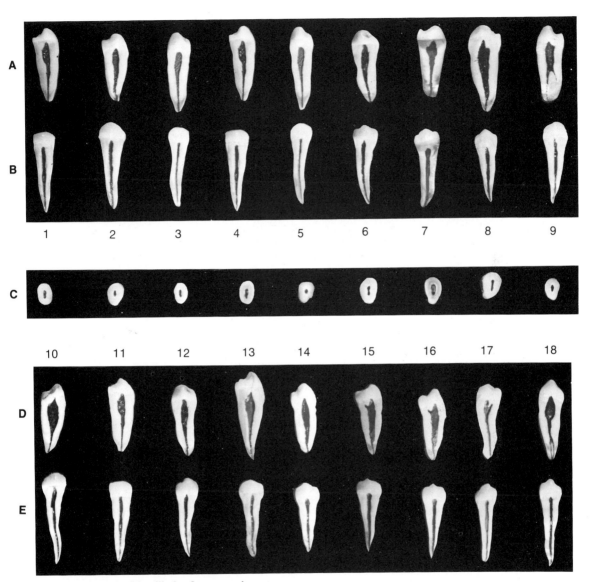

Figure 6–4 Mandibular first premolar.

A, Buccolingual cross section, exposing the mesial or distal aspect of the pulp cavity. This aspect will not show in a dental radiograph taken in the usual manner.

B, Mesiodistal cross section, exposing the buccal or lingual aspect of the pulp cavity.

C, Cervical cross section. A transverse cut at the cementoenamel junction, exposing the pulp chamber. These are the openings to root canals that will be seen at that level.

D, Buccolingual cross section, exposing the mesial or distal aspect of the pulp cavity.

E, Mesiodistal cross section, exposing the buccal or lingual aspect of the pulp cavity.

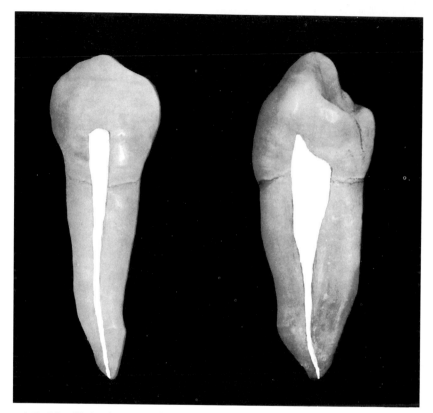

Figure 6–5 Mandibular first premolar, buccal aspect and mesial aspect. Normal pulp cavity forms are painted on the tooth surfaces as they might appear in their relative cross sections. Note the comparison between the spacing and form of the pulp chamber portion in the crown of one aspect as distinguished from that of the other. Viewed from the buccal aspect, the pulp chamber portion of the pulp cavity is narrow and the root canal becomes even narrower as it tapers toward the apical end of the root; viewed from the mesial aspect, the pulp chamber portion is pointed toward the tip of the well-formed buccal cusp of the crown and is quite wide in a buccolingual direction as it copies the level of the linguo-occlusal surface. The root canal tapers gradually but holds a substantial width buccolingually until it reaches midroot approximately. It narrows rapidly here, continuing much more constricted on its way to the apical end of the root (Fig. 6–4, *A*).

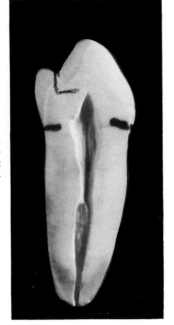

Figure 6–6 A buccolingual section of a mandibular first premolar. The cervical markings indicate the proximity of the cementoenamel junction to the pulp chamber. The occlusal markings suggest an estimated cut for cavity preparation and its proximity to the buccal pulp horn accommodation in the pulp chamber.

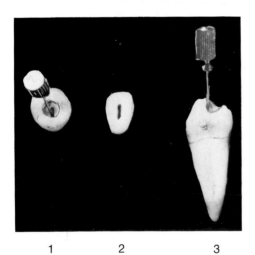

1   2   3

Figure 6–7 Mandibular first premolar. 1, Occlusal view of occlusal opening necessary to facilitate entrance of root canal instruments. 2, The root outline and pulp chamber opening to be found at the level of cementoenamel junction. 3, Profile view buccolingually, showing relationship of the alignment of the instrument to the opening in the crown. The cusp of the mandibular first premolar leans lingually so that it is almost centered over the root. The occlusal opening must approach the cusp tip in order to allow easy access to instruments. In this respect this tooth is similar to the mandibular canine.

Figure 6–8 Mandibular first premolar. Compare this figure with Figure 6–7. 1, A small opening made in the central groove of the occlusal surface will not allow access to the root canal because of the angulation of the occlusal surface with long axis of the root. 2, A cut-out that indicates the minimum of occlusal access permissible. 3, Even with the generous opening into the occlusal surface, care will be required in approaching the apical third of the root.

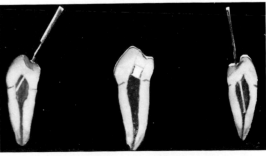

1   2   3

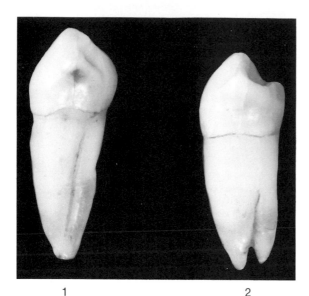

1   2

Figure 6–9 Mandibular first premolar—two specimens with anomalous roots.

In the introduction to this chapter, the statement was made that in diagnosis, the endodontist must be aware of the possibility of malformation of mandibular first premolar roots. Two tooth specimens with anomalous involvement are shown (see also Fig. 6–10).

1, This specimen presents the appearance of two roots fused into one with a deep developmental groove most of the root length.

2, This specimen has a smooth, well-formed root for over half its length below the cementoenamel junction. Then a distinct bifurcation gives the root two apical portions.

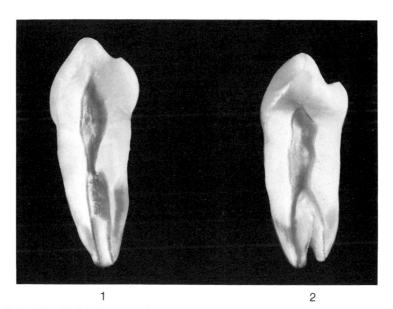

1   2

Figure 6–10 Mandibular first premolar, buccolingual dissections.

These two specimens are the same teeth placed in the same relationship as those shown in Figure 6–9. The buccolingual dissections demonstrate variations in the pulp cavity forms when compared with specimens with normal root development (see Fig. 6–4, A, D).

1, This specimen has a normal pulp cavity within the crown and for about half the root length. Then a branching takes place, amounting to two narrow root canals approximately parallel and ending in two apical foramina. A small piece was lost during the preparation that marked the point of root canal division. However, the original root canal design is apparent.

2, This specimen is odd in every way when its development is compared with the normal pulp cavity formation. Its pulp chamber lacks normal extension into the crown portion. Also, the midroot portion remains wide for at least half the root length apically. Then there is a clean division of the root canal into two branches with abrupt angulations before continuing to form two foramina at the apical ends of the divided root.

Needless to say, unexpected pulp cavity formations like these two examples make endodontic treatment difficult. If the diagnosis of such a situation were suspected before treatment, the operator would have an opportunity to waive responsibility if endodontic treatment were to fail.

118

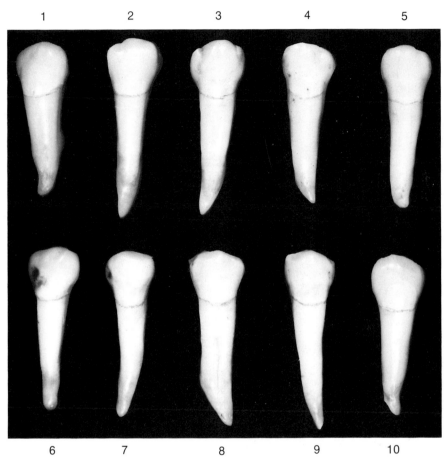

Figure 6–11 Root form of the mandibular second premolar, buccal aspect. The cervical portion of the root is usually broader than that of the mandibular first premolar. The bulky root of generous length has a more gradual taper from the cementoenamel junction to a blunt root end or a root ending in a "sudden point." (Compare 5 with 4.) The root is broader in all directions and usually longer than the first premolar root.

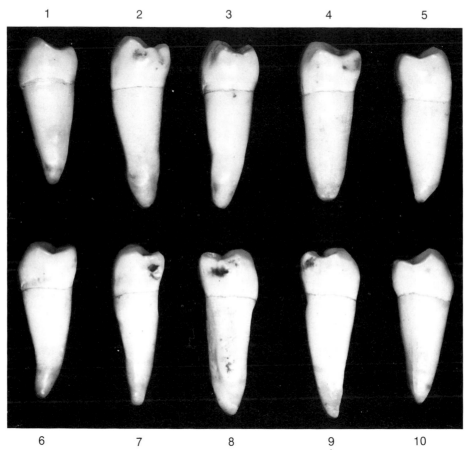

Figure 6–12   Root form of the mandibular second premolar, mesial aspect. Because the crown is wider buccolingually than the mandibular first premolar, the root of the mandibular second premolar follows suit. The root is quite wide buccolingually, ending in a blunted apical portion in most cases. The root tapers toward the apex in a gradual manner, keeping the root width below its midpoint. There are exceptions, of course, as in all anatomical areas (6 and 10).

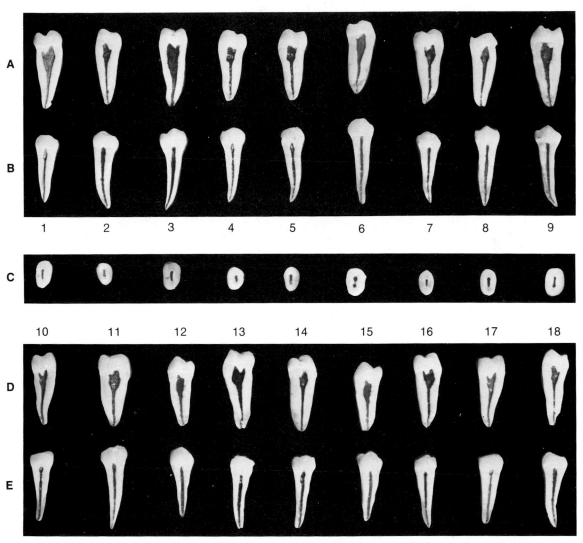

Figure 6–13 Mandibular second premolar.

A, Buccolingual cross section, exposing the mesial or distal aspect of the pulp cavity. This aspect will not show in a dental radiograph made with standard technique.

B, Mesiodistal cross section, exposing the buccal or lingual aspect of the pulp cavity.

C, Cervical cross section. A transverse cut at the cementoenamel junction, exposing the pulp chamber. These are the openings to root canals that will be seen at that level.

D, Buccolingual cross section, exposing the mesial or distal aspect of the pulp cavity.

E, Mesiodistal cross section, exposing the buccal or lingual aspect of the pulp cavity.

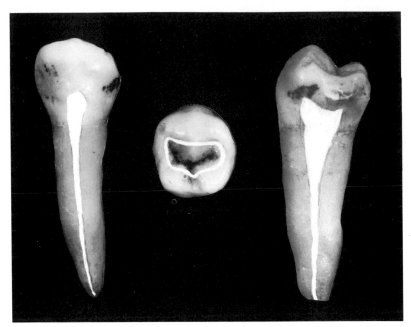

Figure 6–14 Mandibular second premolar, buccal, occlusal, and distal aspects.

Normal pulp cavity form is painted on the buccal and distal tooth surfaces as they might appear in their related cross sections. Because this tooth has a working occlusal surface with central developmental grooves directly over the pulp chamber, an outline is painted on an occlusal view of this tooth suggesting the periphery of an occlusal opening required to gain proper access for endodontic treatment.

The design of the pulp cavity as it would appear in a mesiodistal cross section follows, as usual, an approximation of the outline of crown and root, only in miniature. This is true also of the pulp cavity design as it would appear in a buccolingual cross section. Since the crown and cervical portion of the root of the mandibular second molar show considerable bulk from the distal or mesial aspect, the mass of tissue in vivo from this aspect would follow suit as portrayed by the painted photo on the right.

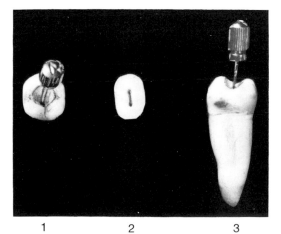

1   2   3

Figure 6–15 The mandibular second premolar.

1, Occlusal view of canal instrument entering the root canal occlusally. Note the size of the opening necessary to properly approach the pulp chamber.

2, Cross section of this tooth at the cervical line that exposes the pulp chamber.

3, Profile view buccolingually, showing the angle at which the instrument enters the root canal. Compare this picture with its counterpart showing the mandibular *first* premolar in Figure 6–7. See also Figure 6–19.

Figure 6–16 Mandibular second premolar. Actual cross sections. 1, A small opening in the center of the occlusal surface will leave undercuts in the pulp chamber roof. 2, A window in the side of the specimen indicates the width of opening necessary to obliterate undercuts. 3, A probe placed over the photo to show the straight approach possible when dealing with the mandibular second premolar. Nevertheless, it must be noted that the lingual wall only is in line with the center of the occlusal surface.

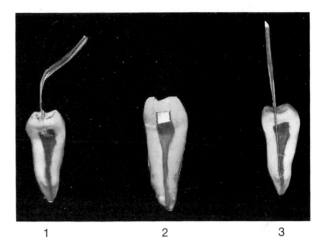

1   2   3

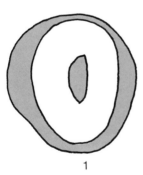 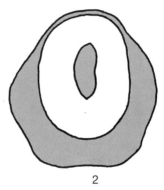

1   2

Figure 6–17 A comparison of tooth form proportions of mandibular first and second premolars.
1, Mandibular first premolar, occlusal aspect.
2, Mandibular second premolar, occlusal aspect.
The overall proportions of each tooth crown are shown in silhouette. The outline of cervical portions of each tooth are superimposed in white over the shaded crowns in the relationship they would assume as to dimensional outlines from occlusal aspects. Pulp cavities are also shaded and placed in good relations with occlusal surfaces.

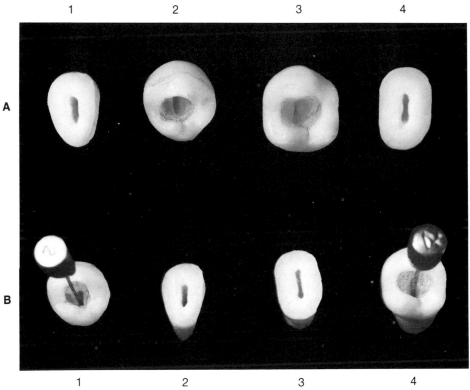

Figure 6–18   A continued comparison of the anatomical characteristics of mandibular first and second premolars—direct occlusal aspects, cervical cross sections, pulp chamber floors.
  A, 1 and 2, Mandibular first premolar; 3 and 4, mandibular second premolar.
  B, 1 and 2, Mandibular first premolar; 3 and 4, mandibular second premolar.

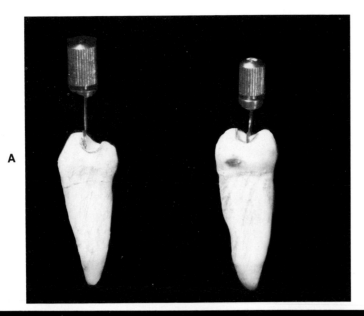

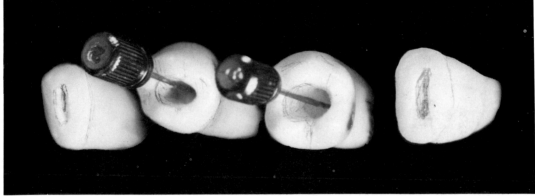

Figure 6–19 The approach to pulp cavities with instruments in mandibular first and second premolars.

A, A profile view of both mandibular premolars with root canal instruments inserted well into the canals. The first premolar is on the left; the second premolar on the right. Note the relationship to buccal cusps and occlusal centers. In order to follow the canal, the instrument placed in the first premolar is forced against the buccal periphery of the occlusal opening (see Fig. 6–7). The instrument placed in the mandibular second premolar is centered in the occlusal opening without strain (see Fig. 6–15).

B, Odd angles in perspective of both mandibular premolar specimens. The specimens shown are placed so that the viewer may get a "close up" of the relationship of instruments to tooth crowns as seen at an angle from an occlusal aspect. Also, there has been some enlargement. Alongside each specimen with instruments is a cervical cross section of a related type. The cervical sections demonstrate that pulp cavities are centered in the root forms. Therefore, the variations in the instrument approach to the crown openings is dependent upon the alignment of crown to root. *The two mandibular premolars differ considerably in this respect.*

CHAPTER 7

Maxillary Second and Third Molars

In form and alignment the maxillary second and third molars adapt themselves to their preceptor, the maxillary first molar. The shapes of crowns and roots follow a similar pattern with adaptations in dimensions to suit their requirements as molars that are related in the upper arch.

Anyone interested in these teeth from the endodontic point of view will be concerned with root formations. In this area, the variations from the first molar form can be considerable. Subsequent descriptions of these comparisons with accompanying illustrations will be presented later in this chapter.

In contrast to earlier years during which foolish attitudes about the value of natural teeth prevailed, the public is now quite interested in the conservation of maxillary second and third molars. By far, the patients requiring endodontic service on maxillary second and third molars are among those in middle life or older. Often these teeth are useful as occlusal supports, either through assumption of their accustomed duties in the dental arch or by acting as abutment anchorages for fixed and removable appliances.

Still, the need for possible endodontic treatment among younger patients cannot be ruled out because some young people are vulnerable to the ravages of dental caries. Therefore, as in other chapters, a calcification table is provided and can be reviewed in association with the Schour-Massler chart. Figure 7–1 presents three sections of the chart, showing tooth development at 12 years (plus or minus 6 months), 15 years (plus or minus 6 months), and 21 years of age. The latter section depicts complete development of all second and third molars.

The location of maxillary second and third molars in the mouth makes endodontic treatment difficult. However, these teeth favor the operator in this way: when contrasted with the first molars, which are positioned more conveniently but are older in development, it will be discovered that root canals are more open

126

and accessible in second and third molars because of the age differential. It will be remembered that second molars are approximately 6 years younger than first molars in the same mouth; the roots may not be complete until 15 years of age or more; the age of third molars ranges from 18 years to 25 years before roots are likely to be complete.

Formerly, third molars were overlooked as valuable candidates for endodontic treatment. Today, this attitude has changed; because of the chronological lag in development, the endodontist has found it an advantage to be experienced in the manipulation of instruments and materials in "younger" pulp cavities, especially as offered by third molars. The open canals and their accessibility counterbalance uncertainties that might be associated with the variance in pulp cavity anatomy.

MAXILLARY SECOND MOLAR

CALCIFICATION OF THE MAXILLARY SECOND MOLAR

First evidence of calcification	2½ to	3 years
Enamel completed	7 to	8 years
Eruption	12 to	13 years
Root completed	14 to	16 years

CROSS-SECTIONAL ANATOMY: DESIGN OF PULP CAVITIES (Fig. 7–5, *A, B, C, D, E*)

Buccolingual Cross Section (Fig. 7–5, *A, D*)

The form of any pulp cavity will be affected by the shape of the tooth; therefore, in order to describe the cavity as presented by the buccolingual cross section of the maxillary second molar, a review of the tooth form is required. The review is simplified by comparing the second molar with the maxillary first molar. Biologically, all first molars serve as model patterns for the remaining molars, both maxillary and mandibular. When well formed, the buccal roots of maxillary second molars are straighter and closer together than those of the maxillary first molars. There is a greater tendency toward fusion of roots, but most second molars will possess a lingual root which is entirely separate and well developed (Fig. 7–5, *A*, 1, 2, 3, 6). The second molar has a crown at least as wide buccolingually as the first molar; therefore, the pulp chamber will be of generous proportions buccolingually also. The buccolingual cross section shows that the mesiobuccal root canal is less complicated than that of the first molar and, therefore, it is more favorable for endodontic treatment. As a rule, the mesiobuc-cal root of the maxillary second molar will house only one root canal. Anomalies are found, however (Fig. 7–5, *A*, 5, 7). The pulp chamber roof from this angle exhibits the form that was necessary to enclose the pulp horns in vivo.

Mesiodistal Cross Section (Fig. 7–5, *B*, *E*)

It may be noted in the illustration of mesiodistal cross sections of maxillary second molars that the design of pulp chamber and root canals compares favorably with those of the maxillary first molars in this cross section. The buccal roots may not spread apart as much, and there may be a greater tendency for the fusion of roots. The pulp chamber is constricted from this angle, but pulp horn formation is still much in evidence.

Cervical Cross Section (Fig. 7–5, *C*)

The cervical cross section of the maxillary second molar will reflect the more extreme angulation of the second molar crown form when compared with the maxillary first molar. The mesiobuc-cal line angle is more acute, and the distobuccal line angle is more obtuse (Fig. 7–5, *C*, 2, 5). The outline of the pulp chamber will reflect this form. The location of pulp canals will be noted as follows: the mesiobuccal canal will seem far buccal, as well as mesial, following the form of the acute mesiobuccal angulation (Fig. 7–9); the distobuccal canal more nearly approaches the mid-point distally in the floor of the pulp chamber between the mesio-buccal canal and the lingual canal. The latter assumes the typical locale (Fig. 7–10).

Midroot Sections

Although the roots of the maxillary second molar seem less well developed than those of the first molar, in most cases they are reasonably well formed and separated (Fig. 7–5, *C*, 6, 7, 9). The midroot sections will show small openings of root canals at this point; nevertheless, these are distinct openings. If the mesiobuccal root happens to be as broad and flat as that of the first molar, it may have two canals (Fig. 7–5, *C*, 8). This specimen shows max-illary second molar roots that developed close together, with some fusion having taken place (see also Fig. 7–5, *C*, 7; *A*, 5, 7).

MAXILLARY THIRD MOLAR

CALCIFICATION OF THE MAXILLARY THIRD MOLAR

First evidence of calcification	7 to 9 years
Enamel completed	12 to 16 years
Eruption	17 to 21 years
Root completed	18 to 25 years

CROSS-SECTIONAL ANATOMY: DESIGN OF PULP CAVITIES (Fig. 7–18, *A, B, C, D, E*)

Maxillary third molars vary so much in development that there will be no attempt here to describe the usual specific cross sections in detail. Nevertheless, a sample of cross sections displayed in the same manner and number for comparison with the cross sections of neighboring maxillary molars is indicated. These can be studied in Figure 7–18. When the development and eruption of the maxillary third molar can be compared with the other maxillary molars, this tooth will have the appearance of being a smaller and weaker maxillary second molar. The crown will be triangular rather than quadrilateral; the roots will be shorter and more curved than those of the second molar, and in many cases they will show a tendency toward fusion into the equivalent of one tapered root (Fig. 7–14, 2, 5, 6). These descriptions include most normally developed maxillary third molars, but the statement that they apply to the majority of these teeth could be erroneous. To the endodontist, biologically, the maxillary third molar has one fact in its favor—it is 8 or 9 years younger than the first molar. Normally, the pulp chambers and root canals of the third molar submit to treatment more readily as a consequence. However, this does not take into consideration the likelihood of having to deal with malformations so often found during the clinical examination. Many maxillary third molars will depart from the normal in crown and root formation. Naturally, in those cases the pulp cavities will depart from the normal also (Figs. 7–21, 7–22, and 7–23, *B*). Although third molars as a class have been condemned generally by both the dental profession and the laity, they must not be condemned without "trial and investigation." Many a third molar, properly nurtured, has been an asset much appreciated by everyone concerned, and especially so by their hosts in the years following successful treatment.

SUMMARY—MAXILLARY SECOND AND THIRD MOLARS

Maxillary second and third molars can be of value, especially later in life, when the stabilization of jaw relations may become a problem. At times they are needed as occlusal supports and as anchorage for appliances when most of the original dependencies have been lost. Sometimes the maxillary second and third molars aid an individual in holding on to the "last vestiges of youth," as represented by his original jaw relations and by the remainder of occlusal stability which could assure some permanence of facial characteristics.

Fortunately, most people are interested in conserving their personal attributes, which include any teeth that can be saved. No longer do they take the position that "sooner or later they will lose all their teeth, so why put off the evil day! Have the teeth extracted and get used to dentures while still young and adaptable!" If people taking this attitude had an opportunity to find out what experienced dentists and people associated with the dental profession planned for themselves under the same circumstances, they would come to a much different conclusion! Second and third molars in both jaws are at times the only teeth left (except perhaps the lower anterior teeth) that remain as dental assets. Sometimes, also, successful endodontic treatment is the only measure that can be depended upon to ensure the status quo in the dental arch.

Although the location of maxillary second and third molars makes endodontic treatment of them difficult, at the same time, they may permit access to pulp chambers and root canals with more facility than do teeth anterior to them, because they are years younger chronologically.

If, in any one case, there are contemporary posterior teeth in the opposite jaw with which they can occlude, it would be difficult to place a value on maxillary second and third molars capable of being saved. The establishment of occlusal levels posteriorly lends permanency to jaw relations and helps to ensure oral health.

MAXILLARY SECOND MOLARS

Figure 7–2 Maxillary second molars—root form, buccal aspect.

Ten representative specimens of the maxillary second molar, with special emphasis on root form and development. The two buccal roots are featured from this aspect.

The buccal roots have about the same length. They have a tendency to stay together and to lean distally. Occasionally the buccal roots will spread similar to the maxillary first molar (specimen 1). All the second molar roots are of good length, exceeding the first molar in the same mouth on occasion.

Sometimes the bending of long roots distally will place their apical ends beyond the distal outline of the tooth crown (specimens 2, 6, 8).

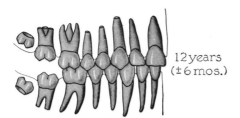

12 years
(±6 mos.)

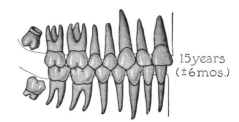

15 years
(±6 mos.)

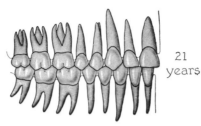

21
years

Figure 7–1 Development and maturation of the maxillary second and third molars. These three divisions of the chart on the development of the human dentition by Schour and Massler illustrate the development of maxillary second and third molars with associated chronology extending from 12 to 21 years. The maturation of the root forms will be of interest to those involved in the endodontic treatment of them. (From The development of human dentition. J.A.D.A., *28*:1153–1160, 1941, by I. Schour and M. Massler, University of Illinois College of Dentistry.)

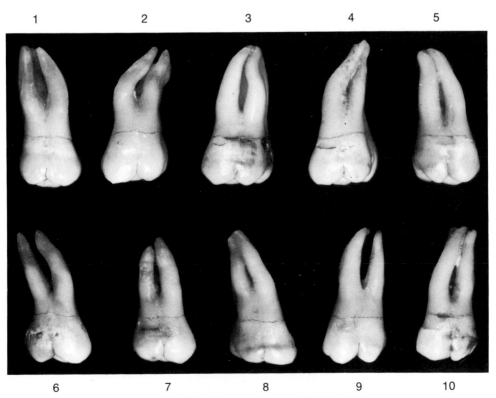

Figure 7–2 *See opposite page for legend.*

131

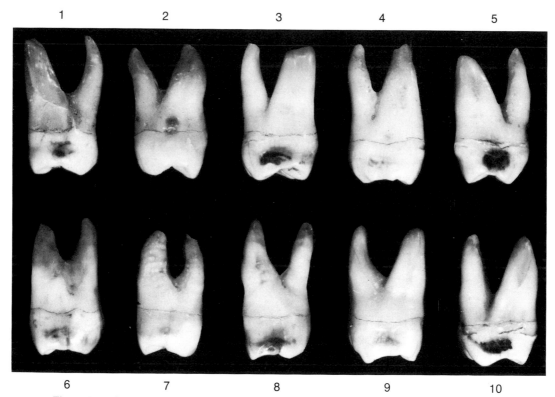

Figure 7–3 Maxillary second molars—root form, mesial aspect.

Ten representative specimens (same as shown in Fig. 7–2) of the maxillary second molar with emphasis on root form and development. The mesiobuccal root and the lingual root are featured from this aspect. These two roots are not quite as well formed as maxillary first molars, and they spread apart less. Again, specimen 1 in the illustration is the exception. Since the mesiobuccal root is less generous in formation buccolingually, the pulp cavity formation will be simpler also when making comparisons with the maxillary first molar. There can be exceptions, of course (Fig. 7–5, *A*, 5, 7). As a rule, the mesiobuccal root will harbor a single root canal.

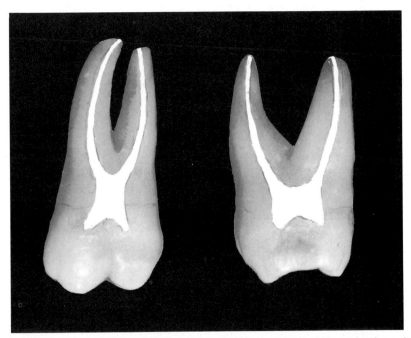

Figure 7–4 Maxillary second molar, buccal aspect and mesial aspect. Normal pulp cavity form is painted on the tooth surfaces as they might appear in their relative cross sections. The cavity form of the maxillary second molar compares favorably with that of the maxillary first molar. Any variation may be attributed to adaptations to the second molar form which has the following individualities when compared with the first molar: the crown is more rhomboidal from the occlusal aspect; buccal roots tend to be closer together with less flair; the buccolingual measurement of the mesiobuccal root is less, which tends to confine the root canal design to one canal in that root in most cases (Figs. 7–5, *A, D,* and 7–8).

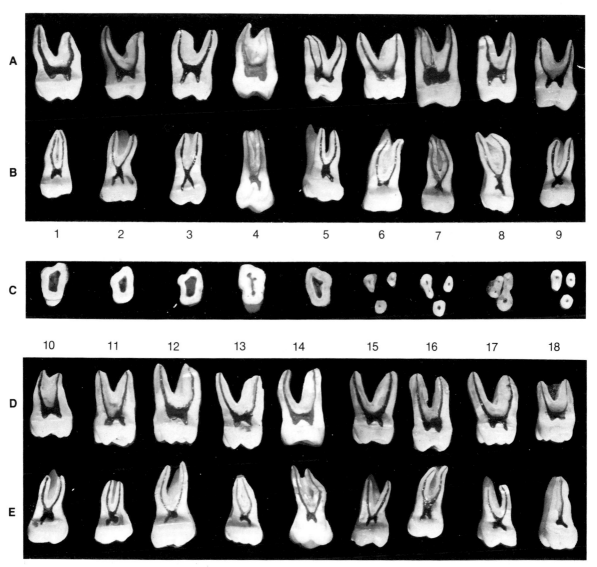

Figure 7–5 Maxillary second molar.

A, Buccolingual cross section, exposing the mesial or distal aspect of the pulp cavity. This aspect does not show in standard dental radiographs.

B, Mesiodistal cross section, exposing the buccal or lingual aspect of the pulp cavity.

C, Five transverse cross sections at cervical line and four transverse sections at midroot.

D, Buccolingual cross section, exposing the mesial or distal aspect of the pulp cavity.

E, Mesiodistal cross section, exposing the buccal or lingual aspect of the pulp cavity.

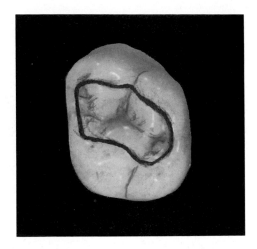

Figure 7–6 Maxillary second molar—occlusal opening suggested for convenient access to the pulp chamber and root canals.

When instruments are placed in the initial directional paths for root canals in this tooth, the shafts will sometimes approach the periphery of the occlusal opening, even when it is enlarged as pictured. When placed in buccal root canals, for instance, the handle end of the instruments may approach the marginal ridge areas of the occlusal surface (Figs. 7–7 and 7–9, 1).

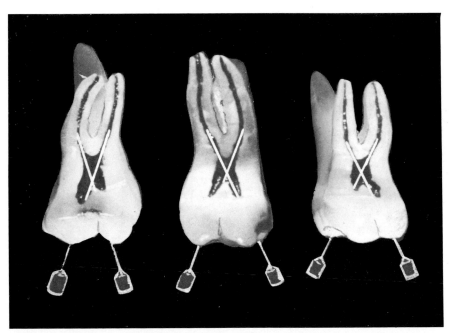

Figure 7–7 Maxillary second molar, mesiodistal cross section. Three well-formed specimens of the maxillary second molar, with simulated canal instruments placed at the angle required to enter the buccal root canals. The rather extreme angle is required to traverse the cervical third of the roots; then the instruments must have flexibility sufficient to allow curvature to be negotiated on the way to the apical ends of the buccal roots. This illustration compares favorably with Figures 2–11 and 2–12, which depict the same aspect of the maxillary first molar. Plainly, the occlusal opening required for instrument approach should be generous, as shown in Figure 7–6.

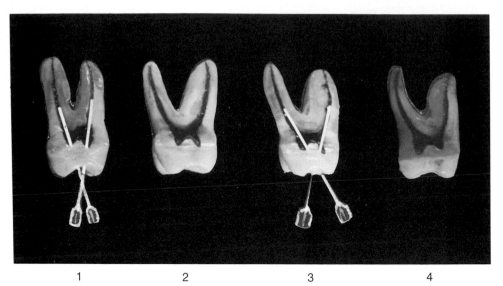

1   2   3   4

Figure 7–8 Maxillary second molar, buccolingual cross sections.

Four typical specimens of the maxillary second molar with the mesiobuccal and lingual roots sectioned in a buccolingual direction. They show little variation in pulp cavity form when all are compared. Specimen 1 shows less separation of roots; this form allows a straighter approach to root canals from this aspect. Specimen 3 is probably more typical with the instrument approach comparable to that required for the maxillary first molar (Fig. 2–19, *A* and 2–20).

It will be noted that all four specimens show single root canals in the mesiobuccal roots from this aspect. This form is a characteristic of the maxillary second molar; remember, the maxillary first molar was considered erratic in this regard. However, the endodontist must always look for exceptions to all anatomical "rules."

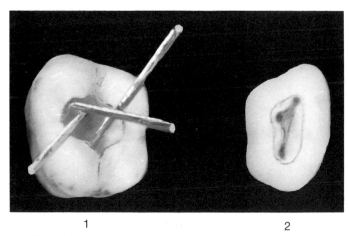

1   2

Figure 7–9 Maxillary left and right second molars—pulp chamber approach to root canals.

1, Occlusal aspect of a maxillary *left* second molar with the occlusal opening suggested for the proper access to the pulp chamber for root canal instruments. Probes are placed in each of the three canals in the directions they had to take for entry in this specimen.

2, A cervical cross section of a maxillary *right* second molar exposing the pulp chamber that displays the location of entrances to the three root canals. Because of the more acute mesiobuccal line angle possessed by the second molar root trunk, the mesiobuccal root canal opening will be in a more extreme mesiobuccal position than that of the maxillary first molar. The distobuccal and the lingual root canal openings are rather evenly centered on the root base. When all the openings are aligned, they form a distorted "Y."

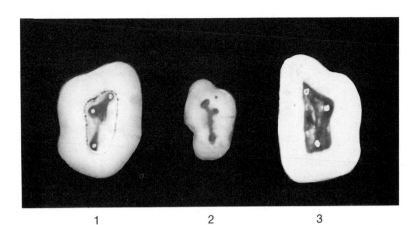

1   2   3

Figure 7–10 Maxillary second molar, cervical cross sections.

The cervical portion of the crown and root of the maxillary second molar is more angular than that of the maxillary first molar. (Compare 1 and 3 of this figure with Figs. 2–14, *B* and 2–29, *A*.) Naturally, this form affects the location of the openings to root canals in the floor of the pulp chamber.

The cervical portions as pictured in 1 and 3 (although enlargements are not identical) show the typical anatomy characteristic of the cervical cross section of the maxillary second molar. The calibration distally is much narrower than the calibration mesially, and the mesiobuccal line angle is more acute than that of the maxillary first molar. Therefore, this figuration must be kept in mind when trying to locate the mesiobuccal root canal, usually far to the mesiobuccal in the floor of the pulp chamber.

Specimen 2 in this figure is a cross section through the root trunk, cut farther root-wise than specimens 1 and 3. It serves as an excellent illustration of the relationship of the roots to the base of the maxillary second molar crown. The root canal openings are centered in root portions; this explains the "distorted Y" design of root canal locations in maxillary molars and especially in the tooth in question, as exemplified by specimen 1.

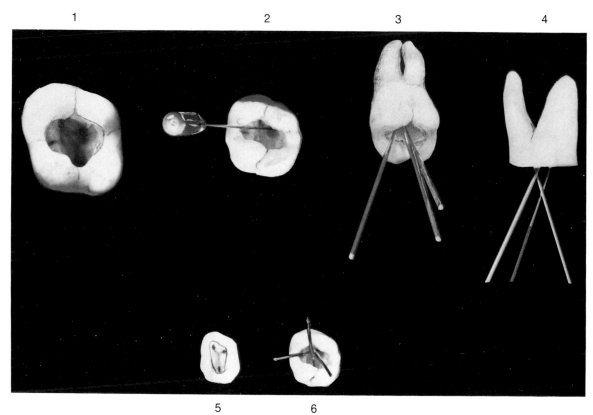

Figure 7–11 Maxillary second molar. 1, Occlusal opening necessary to expose pulp chamber and canals. 2, Extreme angle at which instrument enters distobuccal canal. 3, All three canals have been entered by probers; 3 and 4 emphasize the variation in the angulation of root canals in this tooth. 5 and 6 are photos of second molar pulp chambers: 5, canal locations shown in a cervical cross section; 6, an occlusal view of the open tooth, depicting probe angulations as they enter the three canals.

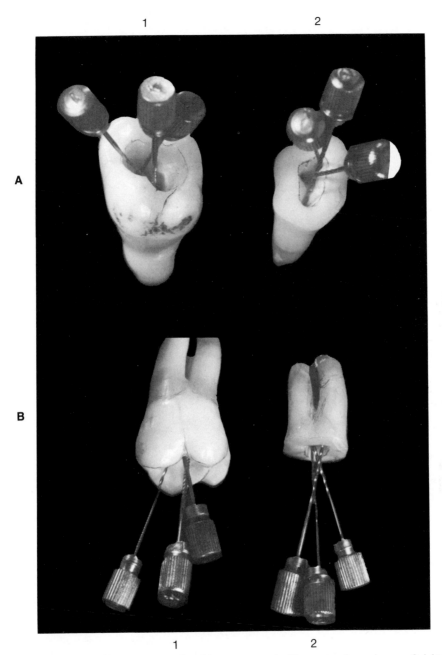

Figure 7–12 Canal instruments pointed into root canals. Two natural specimens of right and left maxillary second molars.

A, 1, Linguo-occlusal aspect of the occlusal opening of a maxillary left second molar with canal instruments placed in the root canals in the directions necessary for entry. 2, A cervical cross section of a right second molar presenting a good view of the root canal entrances in the floor of the open pulp chamber with canal instruments shown entering the canals in their respective alignments. The distobuccal root canal always requires a more extreme angulation for entry.

B, A different camera aspect of the two specimens shown in *A* with the same instruments in place.

A   B

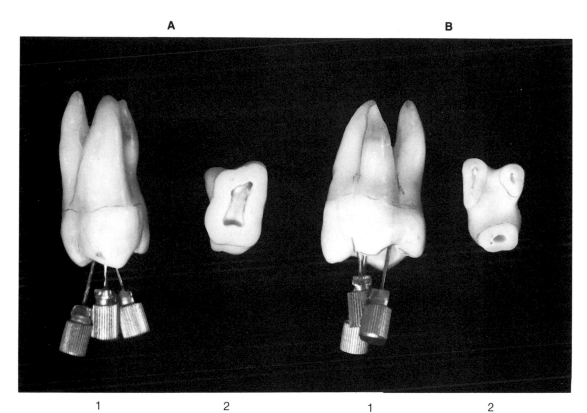

1   2   1   2

Figure 7–13 Maxillary second molar—two aspects of prepared specimens.

A, 1, A mesiobuccal view of the same tooth with instruments in place as that shown in Figure 7–12, *A*, 1; *B*, 1. 2, A cervical cross section of a maxillary second molar of a type more rhomboidal in character than that shown in Figure 7–12, *A*, 2. The exposed pulp chamber is more angular in outline also.

B, 1, A distobuccal view of the same maxillary second molar with instruments in place that allows a change in perspective for comparison with *A*, 1 and with Figure 7–12, *A*, 1; *B*, 1. 2. The specimen shown as *B*, 2 in this figure has been turned over to display the apical aspect of amputated roots at mid-section. The size and shape of root canals will be of interest.

MAXILLARY THIRD MOLARS

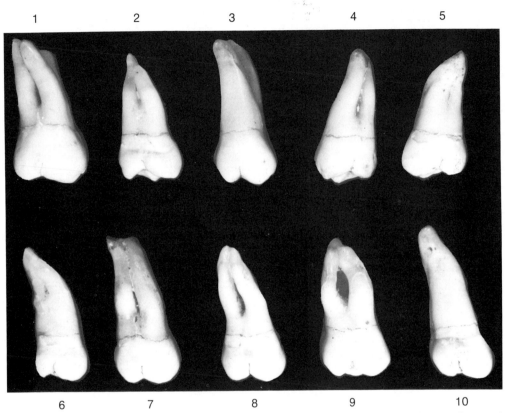

Figure 7–14 Maxillary third molars—root form, buccal aspect. Ten representative specimens of the maxillary third molar with emphasis placed on the root form and development. The tendency in formation is for the fusion of roots, even going so far as to form mechanically what amounts to one pointed and tapered root. Developmental grooving will mark the juncture of formations, but usually little actual spacing between the root forms will be found. As mentioned before, however, third molars in either jaw will show more anomalous variance than any other tooth (Figs. 7–15, 8, 9; 7–16, 10).

1   2   3   4   5

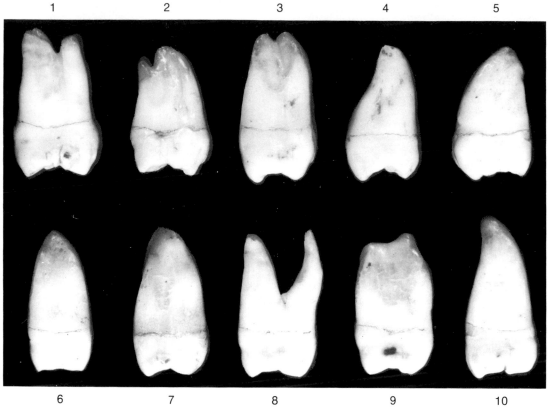

6   7   8   9   10

Figure 7–15 Maxillary third molar root forms, mesial aspect.

These 10 representative specimens of maxillary third molars, with emphasis placed on root form and development, are identical to those displayed in Figure 7–14.

As is often the case, the root forms from *this aspect* do not always show a pointed taper comparable to their buccal or lingual aspects, although some are shaped that way (4, 5, 7, 10). Perhaps as many others show parallel buccal and lingual sides for half or more of root length, rounding off apically to a blunted apical end (1, 3, 6, 9). Demonstrating inconsistency of root form which seems to be in character for third molars, 8 shows well-separated roots from the mesial aspect, very similar in fact to a maxillary second molar.

Figure 7–17 Maxillary third molar, buccal aspect and mesial aspect. The pulp cavity form to be anticipated is painted on the tooth surfaces as they might appear in their relative cross sections. Because of the likelihood of tooth form variation in this tooth, the pulp cavity will vary in direct relation to the developmental changes; therefore, no rules can be established for the anticipation of pulp cavity design in the maxillary third molar. The uncertainty is amplified by the tooth's location in the mouth, even when the alignment is normal.

However, in general, the tooth form development of the maxillary third molar is usually that of a smaller and less perfect maxillary second molar. In addition, there is a tendency toward the fusion of roots, with many of these teeth possessing what amounts to one tapered root (Fig. 7–15, 4, 5, 6). If the root happens to be short and pointed apically, the tooth's retention in the jaw might be questioned. In this respect, the *maxillary* third molar is a poorer risk on the average than the *mandibular* third molar, which can have stronger anchorage and at the same time a more advantageous location for service. All third molars favor the endodontist in one regard; because of their advantage chronologically, the pulp cavities will be more accessible and amenable to manipulation; they will be more open, and secondary dentinal blockage is less likely.

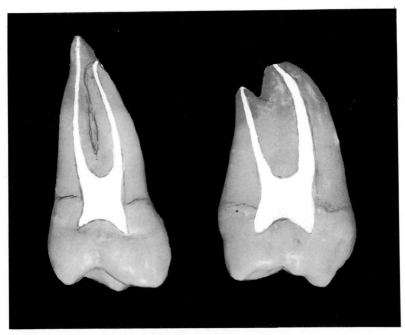

Figure 7–16 Maxillary third molars—12 specimens showing uncommon variations. 1, Very short fused root form. 2, Extremely long roots with extreme distal angulation. 3, Complete fusion of roots with extreme distal angulation. 4, Three roots well separated, crown very wide at cervix. 5, Extreme rhomboidal outline to crown with developmental grooves oddly placed. 6, Overdeveloped mesiobuccal cusp. 7, Crown wide at cervix, with roots perpendicular. 8, Very large crown, poorly developed root form. 9, Complete absence of typical design. 10, Specimen abnormally large, with four roots well separated. 11, Five well-developed cusps, atypical in form. 12, Small specimen, atypical cusp form.

Figure 7–17 *See opposite page for legend.*

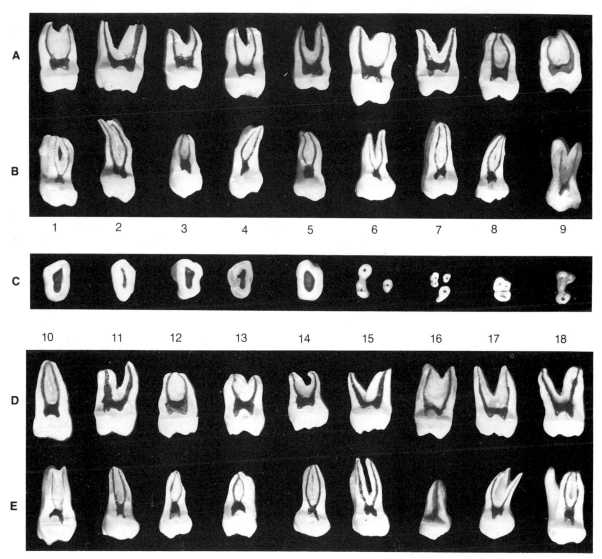

Figure 7–18   Maxillary third molar.
A, Buccolingual cross section, exposing the mesial or distal aspect of the pulp cavity. This aspect will not show on standard dental radiographs.
B, Mesiodistal cross section, exposing the buccal or lingual aspect of the pulp cavity.
C, Five transverse cross sections at cervical line and four transverse sections at midroot.
D, Buccolingual cross section, exposing the mesial or distal aspect of the pulp cavity.
E, Mesiodistal cross section, exposing the buccal or lingual aspect of the pulp cavity.

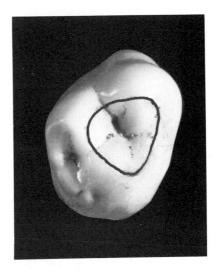

Figure 7–19 Maxillary third molar—occlusal opening for convenient access to the pulp chamber and root canals.

Assuming the three cusp tips of maxillary third molar, which marks the majority, the occlusal opening for convenient access to the pulp chamber and root canals will vary somewhat from the design advocated in other molars. The opening into the center of the occlusal surface will be triangular with rounded corners encompassing the central developmental grooves and the central pit.

In general, the form of the opening is that of a cervical cross section belonging to the type of third molar pictured (Fig. 7–18, *C*, 4). The area of opening will be sufficient to allow instruments to follow the pulp cavity form during endodontic treatment.

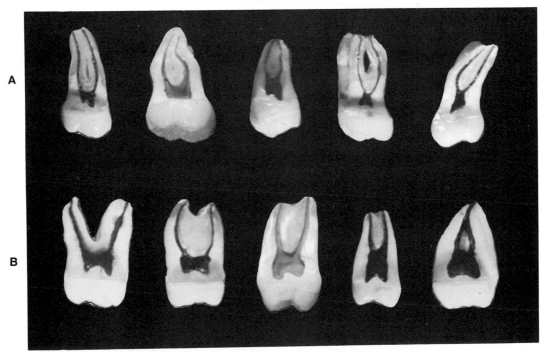

Figure 7–20 Maxillary third molars, mesiodistal and buccolingual cross sections.

A, Mesiodistal cross sections of maxillary third molars chosen at random in order to show a few of the anatomical variations that could be encountered during endodontic manipulations. The angulation at which instruments might enter root canals will vary considerably from this aspect.

B, Buccolingual cross sections of some additional good specimens of the maxillary third molar demonstrate the variance in pulp cavity design from this aspect. The pulp chamber portion is more generous in size, and the continuing root canals are usually wider, improving the possibilities for instrumentation.

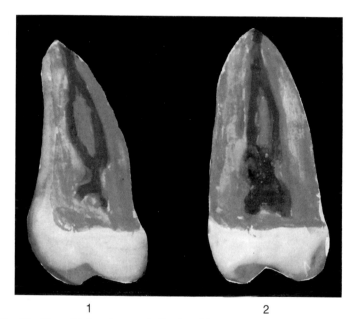

1   2

Figure 7–21 Maxillary third molar, mesiodistal and buccolingual cross sections.

1, Mesiodistal section, right third molar, showing a typical pulp cavity; note the "island" at midroot.

2, Buccolingual section, another right third molar, showing somewhat similar form in a cut that is dissimilar. Generous spacing for pulp tissue is present in both specimens. Note the similarity when these specimens are compared with specimens 1 and 4 in Figure 7–23, *B*).

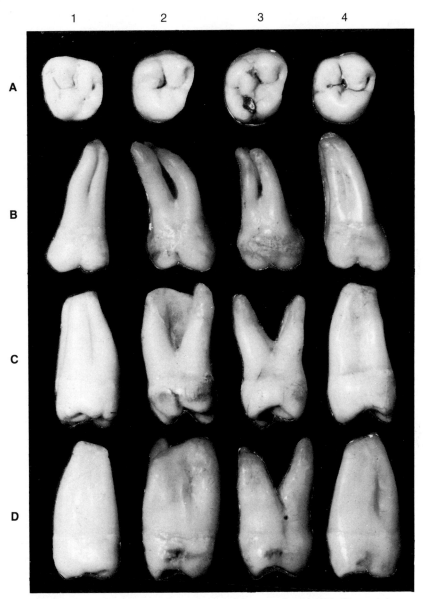

Figure 7–22 Maxillary third molar—four aspects of four specimens. This illustration encompasses four views of four "typical" specimens of the maxillary third molar. The four views were taken before dissections were made to show the pulp cavity design of each one (Fig. 7–23).

A, Top row, straight occlusal aspects of all specimens. Subsequent rows of pictures will keep the same sequence, keeping each tooth in proper perspective. *B*, Buccal aspect. *C*, Distal aspect. *D*, Mesial aspect.

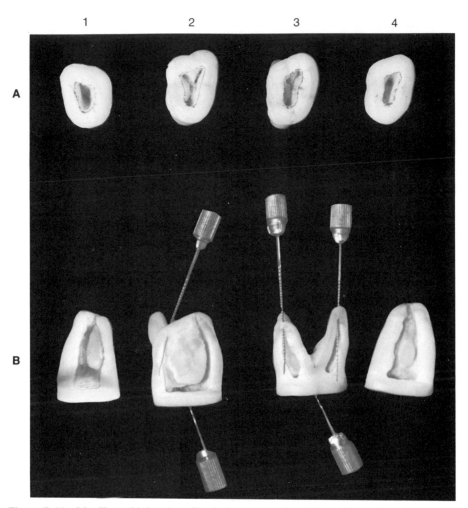

Figure 7–23 Maxillary third molar, Cervical cross sections (*A*) and buccolingual cross sections (*B*).

A, Occlusal aspects of the pulp chambers of the four specimens shown in Figure 7–22. 1 and 4 show a single enlarged entrance to the root canals; 2 and 3 indicate three root canal openings which show some similarity to the usual pulp chamber design expected in maxillary first and second molars. These two specimens also show three individualized root forms in Figure 7–22, taken before dissection.

B, Mesiodistal cross sections of the four specimens in question. 1 and 4 display "island" divisions a short distance from the single pulp chamber openings mentioned under *A*. These obstructions divide each pulp cavity into two root canals which come together apically to form a single foramen. The spacing can be generous and might require the removal of a bulk of tissue as an endodontic measure. The situation shown in specimens 1 and 4 may be suspected in all maxillary third molars with roots fused together (Figs. 7–22, *B*, 1, 4). Specimens 2 and 3 are interesting. These two buccolingual cross sections expose *two root canals*, one *mesiobuccal* and one *lingual*. In specimen 2 the mesiobuccal root and the lingual root are joined. The distobuccal root is individualized (see also Fig. 7–22, *B*, 2; *C*, 2). In the picture of the cross section, the apical foramen of the mesiobuccal canal is marked by the insertion of a No. 1 root canal file. The apical end of the lingual root canal was large enough to show in the dissection. The distobuccal root of the section has a No. 2 root canal reamer inserted well into the root, thereby indicating the relative angulation of the root with its root canal. Specimen 3, another buccolingual cross section, shows clearly wide root canals representative of mesiobuccal and lingual roots in the only third molar in the display grouping which has three roots separated. Two instruments mark the foramina of the mesiobuccal and lingual root canals, and a third root canal instrument is inserted into the distobuccal root, identifying the angulation of its root canal in relation to the other two.

CHAPTER 8

Mandibular Second and Third Molars

The mandibular second and third molars have characteristics in common with the mandibular first molar. The shapes of crowns and roots follow a similar overall design with adaptations in dimensions to suit their functional requirements in the lower dental arch.

The root forms, of course, are of special interest to the endodontist. In this area, one finds some departures from the typical mandibular first molar form. Some observations on this subject are presented on following pages.

In recent years a greater number of dental patients have shown an interest in saving these teeth through endodontic treatment. The lower molars posteriorly have proved to be of priceless value as stabilizers for lower appliances. Also, the ability of all molars to lend occlusal support to the jaw has become widely recognized. The advantages gained by saving the *mandibular* second and third molars may be compared favorably with those mentioned in Chapter 7 under *maxillary* second and third molars. There is one added attraction for the dental operator, however—endodontic manipulation for lower molars is more convenient. Here, too, the age differential, when compared with first molars, makes the mandibular second and third molars a good choice for treatment. Pulp cavities in these teeth are usually more accessible because a second molar is 6 years younger than a first molar, and a third molar is even younger. If the patient is young, the chronology of tooth development must be kept in mind. Treatment of completely calcified roots in such a patient is always more likely to be successful than treatment of immature teeth with unfinished root ends. The Schour and Massler chart section in Chapter 7 (Figure 7–1) provides a graphic presentation of development for both the mandibular second and third molars.

An analysis of the value of *mandibular* second and third molars versus the value of *maxillary* second and third molars would

149

probably favor the former. The loss of either group would be costly, but it is the general consensus of opinion among experienced dental practitioners that complete upper dentures (if it comes to that) can usually be made to be comfortable and successful, whereas the complete loss of tooth anchorage in the lower jaw can be tragic, since most complete lower dentures lack stability.

MANDIBULAR SECOND MOLAR

CALCIFICATION OF THE MANDIBULAR SECOND MOLAR

First evidence of calcification	2½ to 3 years
Enamel completed	7 to 8 years
Eruption	11 to 13 years
Root completed	14 to 15 years

CROSS-SECTIONAL ANATOMY: DESIGN OF PULP CAVITIES (Fig. 8–3, *A, B, C, D, E*)

Buccolingual Cross Section (Fig. 8–3, *A, D*)

Anatomically, the mandibular second molar differs little from the mandibular first molar. The proportions of crown and root are much the same. Therefore, the pulp cavities viewed in cross section will show similarity. Roots of second molars may be straighter, with less spread than first molars; some may have shorter roots, but there is no assurance that any of these differences will be manifest in any one case. However, good radiographs of lower molars are easily obtained and correspond almost exactly to mesiodistal cross sections of these teeth (Fig. 8–3, *B, E*). The length and shape of the roots with pulp chamber and root canals will show clearly.

The buccolingual cross section of the mandibular second molar shows the pulp chamber and pulp canals to be more variable and thus more complicated in form. They are, however, quite similar in most ways to the pulp chamber and cavities of mandibular first molars. A generous pulp chamber that accommodates spaces for well-developed pointed pulp horns, both buccally and lingually, will be evident. Most mandibular second molars will have two canals in the mesial root; some will join in a common apical foramen, whereas others will present one wide flat canal narrowing to a single opening at the root end. (In Fig. 8–3, *A*, compare 1 with 2.) Other well-formed mandibular second molars will have two separate canals in the mesial root that remain divided for the full length of the root, with two separate foramina (Fig. 8–3, *A*, 3, 8; *D*, 12, 14).

Mesiodistal Cross Section (Fig. 8–3, *B, E*)

There will be little to add to the discussion of this cross section for the mandibular second molar because some of these features were covered in the previous section. Except for the tendency toward straighter roots, which may be closer together in some cases, the mandibular second molar looks very much like the mandibular first molar in mesiodistal cross section. Mesial roots will have narrow curved root canals, usually with shorter, straighter, and more open canals in distal roots.

From the endodontic point of view, distal roots with a single, more open canal are usually accessible and penetrable, but mesial root canals may present more of a problem. Therefore, each mandibular second molar must be approached as a likely variation from one treated at a previous session.

Cervical Cross Section (Fig. 8–3, *C*, 1, 2, 3, 4, 5)

The cervical cross section of the mandibular second molar is similar to that of the mandibular first molar. It is not as "square" because the distal portion tapers more. Therefore, the pulp chamber also shows more taper distally. The floor of the pulp chamber will have two openings mesially leading into buccal and lingual root canals in the mesial root and one opening centered distally leading into the single root canal in the distal root.

Midroot Cross Sections (Fig. 8–3, *C*, 6, 7, 8, 9)

Midroot cross sections of the mandibular second molar show little variation. The mesial root will be kidney-shaped, broad buccolingually and narrow mesially. It will present two separate root canals or one canal that is narrow mesiodistally and wide buccolingually. The distal root will be "rounder" than the mesial root; some distal roots may be quite round (Fig. 8–3, *C*, 6, 9). It might be advisable to remind the endodontist that, since people vary genetically, their teeth will vary also. Variations in form and size must be considered when making a clinical diagnosis. The form and dimensions of the parts of a tooth will always have a strong influence on its pulp cavity design.

MANDIBULAR THIRD MOLAR

CALCIFICATION OF THE MANDIBULAR THIRD MOLAR

First evidence of calcification	8 to 10 years
Enamel completed	12 to 16 years
Eruption	17 to 21 years
Root completed	18 to 25 years

CROSS-SECTIONAL ANATOMY: DESIGN OF
PULP CAVITIES (Fig. 8–15, *A, B, C, D, E*)

Mandibular third molars vary greatly in development. Figure 8–15 displays the same number and kinds of cross sections given for the other mandibular molars. These illustrations should be studied and comparisons made.

When the development and eruption of the mandibular third molar are comparable to the other mandibular molars it will closely resemble the second mandibular molar but will look somewhat out of proportion at the same time. The crown may be overly large when associated with the root form; the roots may be short, curved, and inclined toward fusion (Fig. 8–11, *A*, 1, 3, 5).

Cross sections will show all kinds of variations in pulp chambers and root canals. Nevertheless, there are instances in which the retention of this tooth may be of great value to the patient. If the tooth is in good alignment, with favorable retention, it has one factor in its favor. It has the advantage shared by all third molars: it is the youngest by several years of all the individual's other teeth. Therefore, it can be expected that the pulp canals, although odd in formation, might well be reasonably accessible.

A strong mandibular third molar is a good candidate for dental conservation in the mouths of patients who have suffered dental losses. Rather extensive partial appliances can be made more efficient and longer lasting through the use of well-placed mandibular third molars as anchorage abutments. This is especially true when both the right and left molars are available.

They are most valuable as occlusal stabilizers in addition to their function as anchors for saddle extensions in partial appliances.

SUMMARY – MANDIBULAR SECOND AND
THIRD MOLARS

The shapes of crowns and roots of the mandibular second and third molars follow the comprehensive form of the mandibular first molar. The individual dimensions are adapted to suit their functional requirements as indicated by their respective locations in the lower dental arch. These teeth are good candidates for endodontic treatment because of their value as occlusal stabilizers, both in the dental restoration techniques and as anchorage abutments for prosthetic appliances, fixed and removable.

Their chronological age favors their adaptability to endodontic treatment. The application of manipulative treatment in the mandibular second and third molars is simplified because their pulp cavities are more accessible than those of the older teeth anterior to them.

An analysis of the value of these mandibular molars versus the value of maxillary second and third molars would probably weigh in favor of the former. The lower molars have stronger periodontal support, which guarantees a longer life of usefulness. The maxillary second and third molars are more subject to malalignment with consequent periodontal problems.

MANDIBULAR SECOND MOLAR

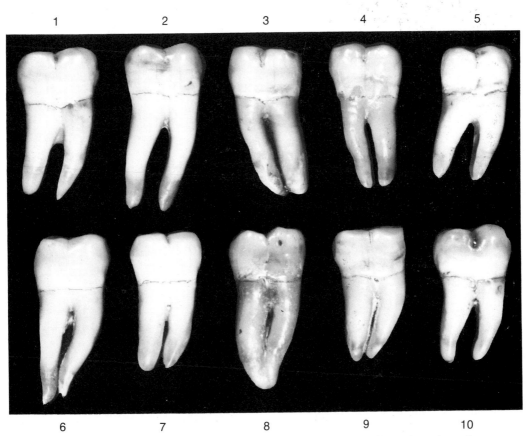

Figure 8–1 Mandibular second molars—root forms, buccal aspect. These 10 good specimens are quite typical of the mandibular second molar. Special emphasis in this illustration is to be placed on the root forms from this aspect. Some second molars have root forms that compare favorably with the mandibular first molar roots (1 and 2). Usually, however, the second molar roots are closer together with a more extreme slant toward the distal (3 and 4). Sometimes the mesial and distal roots are fused apically (8). Quite often the roots of this tooth are longer than the roots of the mandibular first molar in the same mouth.

1   2   3   4   5

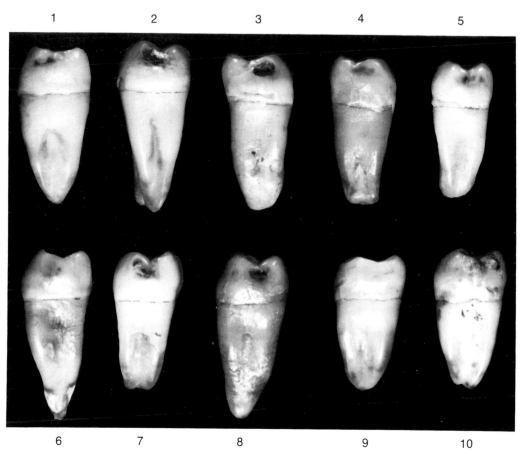

6   7   8   9   10

Figure 8-2 Mandibular second molars—root forms; mesial aspect. These are the same specimens placed in the same rotation as Figure 8-1. Pay particular attention to the root forms as viewed from the mesial aspect. The mesial roots of the mandibular second molars with their overall form are quite similar in design to those of the mandibular first molar. Also, as will be demonstrated in subsequent illustrations, cross sections of second molar roots will reveal pulp cavity anatomy as being similar. Mandibular second molar roots with their housing of root canals, are not quite as consistent in development as the roots of the mandibular first molar. Some of the likely variations were mentioned in Figure 8-1.

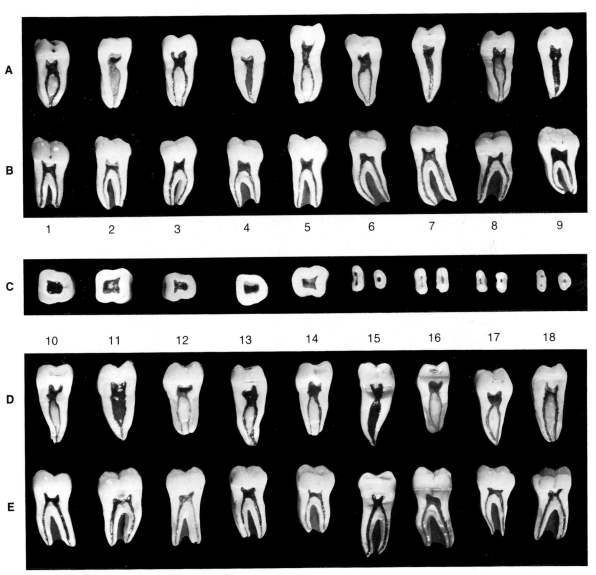

Figure 8–3 Mandibular second molar.

A, Buccolingual cross section, exposing the mesial or distal aspect of the pulp cavity. This aspect does not show on the typical dental radiograph.

B, Mesiodistal cross section, exposing the buccal or lingual aspect of the pulp cavity.

C, Five transverse cross sections at cervical line and four transverse sections at midroot.

D, Buccolingual cross section, exposing the mesial or distal aspect of the pulp cavity.

E, Mesiodistal cross section, exposing the buccal aspect of the pulp cavity.

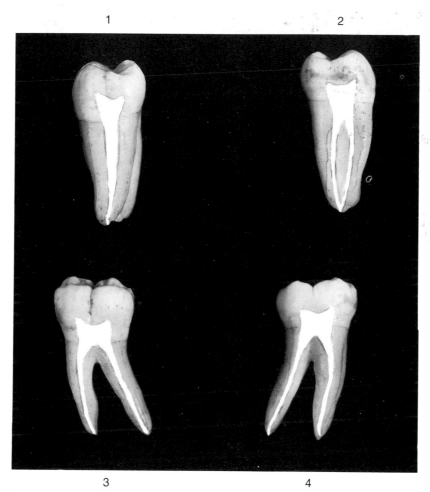

1

2

3

4

Figure 8–4   Mandibular second molar, four aspects. 1, Distal aspect. 2, Mesial aspect. 3, Buccal aspect. 4, Lingual aspect.

The shape of the pulp cavity that seems to be most typical for the mandibular second molar is painted on the various surfaces of the tooth as they might appear in cross sections representing the four aspects. It must be remembered that dental radiographs taken with the usual technique will not present a true picture of pulp cavities as shown in 1 and 2.

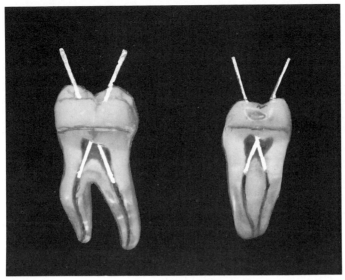

Figure 8–5 Mandibular second molar—the angle of insertion of root canal instruments.

The cross sections of these two specimens show two types of pulp cavity design often encountered. On the left, a mesiodistal cross section of a mandibular second molar with well-separated roots is shown from the buccal aspect. Simulated instruments indicate the angle which must be assumed in order to follow the canal alignment immediately below the pulp chamber. Also, the curvature of the mesial root would require care and dexterity on the part of the operator in order to complete the endodontic treatment. The extreme curvature of the mesial root makes careful application of instruments necessary. As usual, the canal of the distal root is more open and straighter than that of the mesial root.

In the specimen on the right, the mesial root of the mandibular second molar has been dissected in a buccolingual direction. The pulp chamber and the separated canal forms are typical. The canals are curved buccally and lingually, spreading in those directions toward midroot, and then, curving with the root outline, they return to join or approach each other as they form a foramen or foramina (in this case) at the root end. Simulated instruments indicate the angulation required for their entry into the root canals from the pulp chamber floor.

Figure 8–6 Mandibular second molar—root angulation—a pulp chamber floor.

On the left is a nearly ideal specimen of a mandibular second molar with instruments placed in the root canals, showing the alignment of the well-separated roots.

On the right, a cervical cross section of another mandibular second molar specimen is pictured. The tooth was well formed but slightly atypical. The distal portion tapered from the mesial portion, which was typical; however, the floor of the pulp chamber, with its root canal openings, was smoother and plainer than usual.

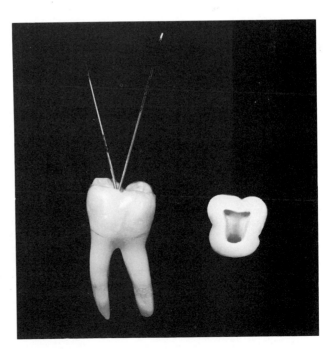

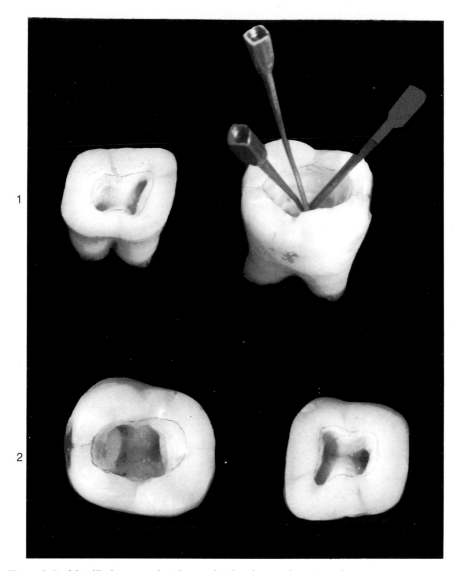

Figure 8-7   Mandibular second molar—pulp chambers and root canals.

1, Left, an angle view occlusally of the pulp chamber floor of a mandibular left second molar with its crown removed. The pulp canal aperture mesially, as usual, is wider than the distal one. The wider opening in this case allows for the entrance of two instruments, indicating separate canals or merely one very wide canal. On the right, a lower right mandibular second molar has instruments placed in the root canals. The angle of the photograph presents a view in perspective of the variance in canal alignments as emphasized by the placement of the probes. The generous occlusal opening in the crown of the tooth allows a well-lighted view and ease in manipulation.

2, A close-up of the two specimens of mandibular second molars in 1, posed in different positions. The right molar is on the left, whereas the left molar is on the right. The straight occlusal view shows very plainly the apertures of root canals in the pulp chamber floors.

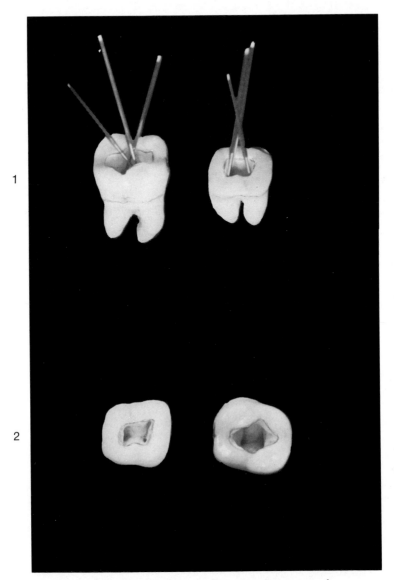

Figure 8–8   Mandibular second molar—two specimens locating root canals.

1, Photographs of two specimens of mandibular second molars showing the wide aperture in the occlusal surface of the complete tooth on the left and the variation in the angulation of instruments placed in three root canal entrances. On the right, a second molar with the crown removed is shown at the same photographic angle as the tooth on the left. Here the pulp chamber is exposed with three instruments in root canal openings. In this specimen, the probes in the mesial root are more nearly parallel than those pictured on the left. This could indicate one wide canal.

2, Occlusal views of the same specimens pictured in 1. It is very difficult to obtain clear photographs of pulp chambers and root canal openings and still get a true picture of the remainder of the tooth specimen in order to register perspective and proportion at the same moment. An experienced operator with a practiced eye would probably accept these pictures as affording a view of pulp chamber and canals superior to the view afforded usually in actual endodontic practice.

1　　　　　　　　2　　　　　　　　3

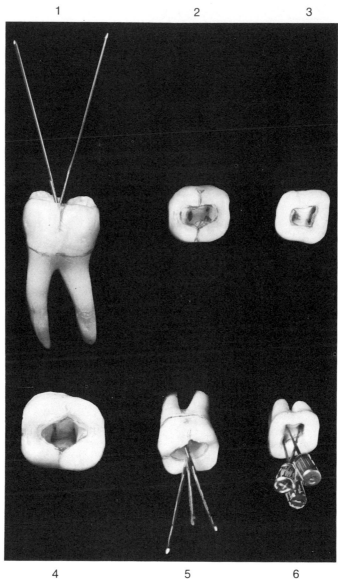

4　　　　　　　　5　　　　　　　　6

Figure 8–9　Mandibular second molar. 1, Buccal view of the mandibular second molar with probes in canals showing the direction of insertion. The picture continues to prove the lack of parallelism existing in multirooted posterior teeth when the directions traversed by pulp canals are pictured. Also, root canals seldom follow a course at right angles to the occlusal surfaces of crowns. 2, Occlusal opening of the left second molar showing easy access to the pulp chamber. 3, A cervical cross section of this molar, which shows graphically in an actual photograph of a natural specimen the shape and location of the canal openings and an anatomically correct outline of the pulp chamber. 4, A close-up of the occlusal opening in the second molar and the approach to the pulp canals. 5, An odd angle of the whole tooth showing the direction taken by probes in the three canals. 6, Instruments placed in the canals with the crown portion of the tooth removed to permit a closer survey of the situation.

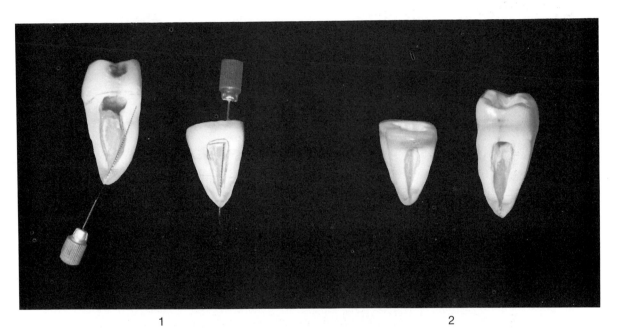

1   2

Figure 8–10   Mandibular second molar, buccolingual root sections.

1, Buccolingual cross sections of the mesial roots of two mandibular second molar specimens. The specimen on the left has the pulp chamber and two more or less parallel root canals exposed, ending in a common apical foramen. A small file penetrates the foramen, which was so tiny that the file was used to locate the undissected tip end of the root. The specimen on the right has had the crown of the tooth removed. This tooth had only *one* wide canal in its *mesial* root. It has the file placed into the open pulp chamber and through the small apical foramen. Both types of mesial root canal design may be said to be commonplace for the mandibular second molar.

2, The same specimens pictured in 1. Each has had its *distal* root dissected in a buccolingual direction. Each one shows the typical shape of root canal (nearly always single) to be expected in the mandibular second molar *distal* root. The canal is narrow mesiodistally and rather wide buccolingually, tapering down to a point locating the apical foramen.

MANDIBULAR THIRD MOLAR

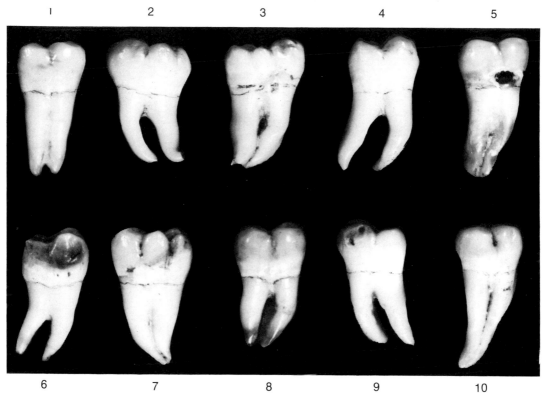

Figure 8–11 Mandibular third molars—root forms, buccal aspect.

These 10 good specimens of the mandibular third molar could be accepted as being representative of this tooth. They would not be regarded as being anomalous in form, although their crown and root forms do not parallel the physiological plans set by molars anterior to them. The specimens on display, however, er, can be accepted as typical with special emphasis placed on the root forms.

Crown forms are typically mandibular molar forms, some appearing oversize when matched with their roots. The root forms, from the buccal aspect, can be grouped into two categories: those that show two roots fused together (3, 5, 10) and those that have two roots well separated in the manner of the more perfectly formed mandibular molar. Generally speaking, the *roots* of the mandibular third molar incline toward dwarfism, while the third molar *crowns* have the opposite tendency. There are exceptions, of course (10). In nearly every instance, the roots are definitely slanted distally. All descriptions of third molar anatomy, *mandibular* or *maxillary,* that attempt to typify them, must be accepted as approximations.

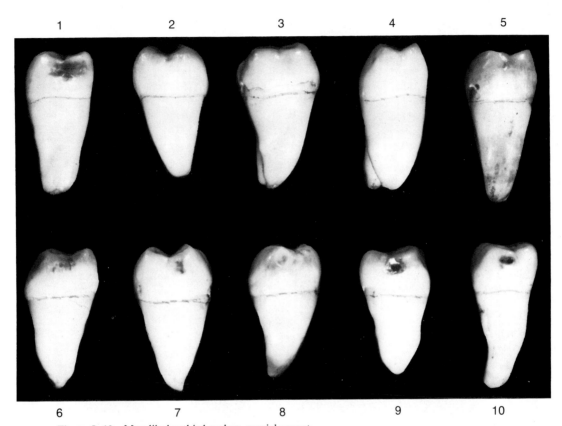

Figure 8–12 Mandibular third molars, mesial aspect.

These 10 specimens are the same teeth posed in the same sequence as in Figure 8–11. From the mesial aspect, these root forms will compare favorably with this aspect of the *mandibular second molar* as pictured in Figure 8–2. They differ in this respect: the roots are somewhat shorter when matched with crown size, and the roots tend to point with rapidly sloping sides.

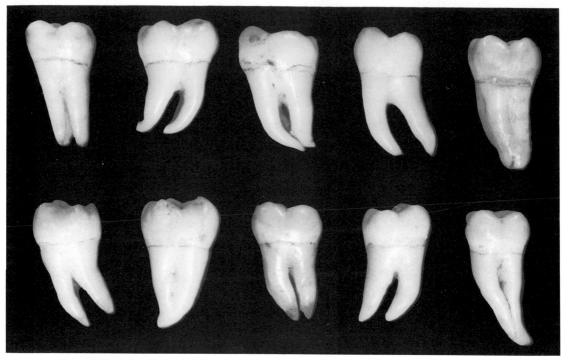

Figure 8–13 Mandibular third molars, lingual aspect. These are the same third molar specimens placed in the same sequence as in Figures 8–11 and 8–12. They are to be compared directly with Figure 8–11, the buccal aspect. Because third molars are inclined to be atypical, a view of these teeth from the lingual as well as the buccal aspect adds perspective in the observation of their root forms.

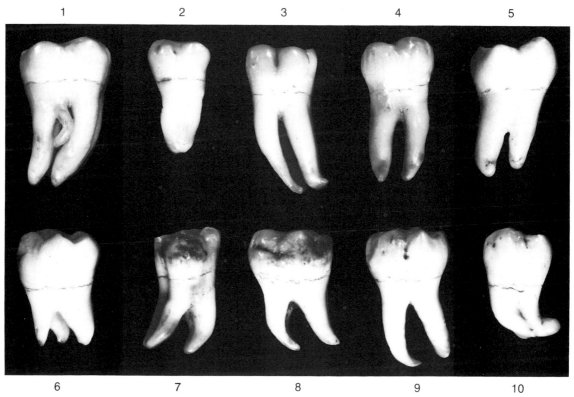

Figure 8–14 *See opposite page for legend.*

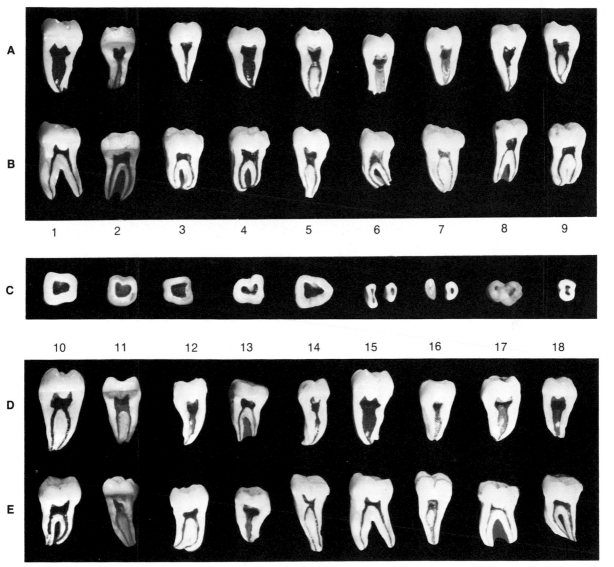

Figure 8–15 Mandibular third molar.

A, Buccolingual cross section, exposing the mesial or distal aspect of the pulp cavity. This aspect does not show on the average dental radiograph.

B, Mesiodistal cross section, exposing the buccal or lingual aspect of the pulp cavity.

C, Five transverse cross sections at cervical line and four transverse sections at midroot.

D, Buccolingual cross section, exposing the mesial or distal aspect of the pulp cavity.

E, Mesiodistal cross section, exposing the buccal or lingual aspect of the pulp cavity.

Figure 8–14 Mandibular third molars—10 specimens showing uncommon variations. 1, Oversized generally, extra root lingually. 2, Dwarfed specimen, odd extra cusp, fused root. 3, Crown resembling first molar, long slender roots. 4, Formation closely resembling second molar. 5, Large crown, malformed roots. 6, Multicusp crown, dwarfed roots. 7, No resemblance to typical functional form. 8, Large crown, dwarfed roots. 9, Odd crown form and root form. 10, Crown long cervico-occlusally, roots fused and malformed.

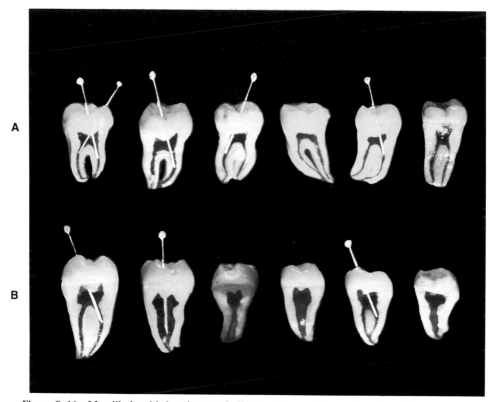

Figure 8–16   Mandibular third molar, mesiodistal sections and buccolingual sections.

A, These mandibular third molar forms are not unusual. The mesiodistal cross sections show considerable variation in pulp cavity formations which of course is typical of most third molars. White lines are projected from some of them, placed to indicate angles at which root canal instruments should be directed in order to enter root canals from this aspect.

B, Six more mandibular third molars demonstrating buccolingual cross sections. It will be noted that from this aspect the cavities seem more open. It must be remembered, however, that although the canals are wider in some instances, they are quite thin and narrow in a mesiodistal direction. These cuts are made into the mesial portion of the tooth, and the "open" canals will match those of the mesial canals in row *A.* The approach with instruments will have to correspond to the more extreme angulations shown in *A* while trying to enter mesial root canals.

CHAPTER 9

Mandibular Incisors

The mandibular incisors are less likely to require endodontic treatment than the other teeth in the mouth. This is fortunate for all concerned because they can present problems. For instance, their small dimensions limit endodontic manipulation; other anatomical limitations are involved also (Figs. 9–11 and 9–12).

These incisors are seldom attacked by dental caries; most people will go through life without ever having a carious cavity in these teeth, even though subject to caries elsewhere in the mouth.

Nevertheless, these teeth are not immune to dental troubles. They are subject to periodontal disorders, and on occasion pulp involvement can be associated with periodontal infection.

Because of the location of the mandibular incisors in the front of the mouth, they are subject to injury from external sources. Remarkably, in an accident they are damaged less often than the maxillary incisors. This may be due to the protection offered the lower teeth by the more prominent upper teeth with their overbite and overjet relationship.

The fact remains that although endodontic service is not required as often for the little incisors, still the service must be made available.

Because they function as a single entity, both mandibular incisors have a similar pulp cavity anatomy. The lateral incisor is slightly wider mesiodistally than the central incisor, and the root may be a trifle longer, but access to and manipulation of the pulp cavity will vary little in the pursuit of endodontic treatment technique.

The following pages will outline some of the anatomical details which must be considered in planning endodontic treatment of the mandibular central and lateral incisors.

MANDIBULAR CENTRAL INCISOR

CALCIFICATION OF THE MANDIBULAR CENTRAL
INCISOR

First evidence of calcification	3 to 4 months
Enamel completed	4 to 5 years
Eruption	6 to 7 years
Root completed	9 years

CROSS-SECTIONAL ANATOMY: DESIGN OF PULP CAVITIES (Fig. 9–4, *A*, *B*, *C*, *D*, *E*)

Labiolingual Cross Section (Fig. 9–4, *A*, *D*)

Although the mandibular central incisor is the smallest tooth in the mouth, it may be noted from this aspect that the labiolingual measurement of crown and root is quite substantial. In fact, the *mandibular central* incisor, along with the *mandibular lateral* incisor, is comparable in this dimension with the *maxillary lateral* incisor.

The pulp cavity, when viewing a labiolingual cross section, seems generous; the spacing is quite broad, conforming to the crown and root outline. This design may be anticipated from this aspect; however, one must remember that the design of the cavity mesiodistally is just the opposite dimensionally—quite thin and narrow. Again, the conformation matches the narrow root dimensions mesiodistally.

Standard dental radiographs will not give a true picture of the labiolingual anatomy. Occasionally, root canals will divide at about midroot, forming two canals (Fig. 9–12, 3), or an "island" may appear, causing a division of the root canal, with the canal duplication joining again before the root end is reached (Fig. 9–14, 5, 6).

Mesiodistal Cross Section (Fig. 9–4, *B*, *E*)

Although the mesiodistal cross section of the mandibular central incisor demonstrates a thin pulp cavity from this aspect, experience proves that ordinarily the root canal will receive the smallest canal files. If care is used, larger instruments may follow so that endodontic technique may progress.

Sometimes, of course, secondary deposit causing severe canal constriction will interfere with penetration (Fig. 9–4, *D*, 16, 18; *E*, 13, 15, 18).

Cervical Cross Section (Fig. 9–4, *C*)

This aspect gives the viewer the proportions of the root trunk of this tooth. Even though the mesiodistal calibration is small, the

labiolingual measurement is large enough to support the tooth when resisting the forces of occlusion. Those forces are applied against the tooth mainly in a labiolingual direction during protrusive and retrusive movements of the jaw.

Figure 9–4, *C* shows that the size and shape of roots of mandibular incisors (mandibular lateral incisors, Fig. 9–8, *C*) will vary to some extent. Before advancing age interferes, the cross sections at the cervical portion will expose pulp cavities as having the same general outline as the periphery of the root formation, and they will be centered within the root.

MANDIBULAR LATERAL INCISOR

CALCIFICATION OF THE MANDIBULAR LATERAL INCISOR

First evidence of calcification	3 to 4 months
Enamel completed	4 to 5 years
Eruption	7 to 8 years
Root completed	10 years

CROSS-SECTIONAL ANATOMY: DESIGN OF PULP CAVITIES (Fig. 9–8, *A, B, C, D, E*)

Labiolingual Cross Section (Fig. 9–8, *A, D*)

The mandibular incisor tends to be *slightly* larger in all calibrations than the mandibular central incisor; therefore, its pulp cavity will vary in size proportionately, but the essential design is the same. The labiolingual cross sections will bear this out. (Compare Fig. 9–4, *A*, with Fig. 9–8, *A*.) The two teeth function in an almost identical manner; therefore, the form and dimensions will be similar, conforming to the same needs. Since the pulp cavity in the mandibular lateral incisor is a little more generous in size, it may prove to be a little more amenable to endodontic treatment.

Mesiodistal Cross Section (Fig. 9–8, *B, E*)

The pulp chamber and canal in this section will demonstrate a slender cavity with even, straight walls for the entire length. It resembles the mandibular central incisor in this respect, but it may appear a little wider and more open. Narrow constrictions and canal blockages would be most likely to show up in this cross section (Fig. 9–8, *E*, 12, 14, 18).

Cervical Cross Section (Fig. 9–8, *C*)

The cervical cross section of the mandibular lateral incisor will show the root canal centered in the root, and before age becomes a problematic factor, the canal is similar in shape to the root periphery. A comparison of root sections will show the root canal to be somewhat larger than that of the mandibular central incisor. Some form variation will also be noticed among numerous specimens. Actually, some cervical sections of the larger specimens will resemble cervical cross sections of small mandibular canines (Fig. 9–8, *C*, 1, 2).

SUMMARY – MANDIBULAR INCISORS

Because the mandibular incisors are less likely to be subject to damage from the usual sources, they will not require endodontic service as often as the other teeth.

Care must be employed when approaching the pulp cavity through the linguoincisal surface because of the anatomical relation of the cavity to the incisal ridge. Flexibility in instrumentation is advocated (Figs. 9–10 and 9–11).

The narrowness of the root forms mesiodistally makes the root canals thin and narrow in that calibration. This constriction must be noted and respected when using canal instruments. The labiolingual dimensions of the pulp cavities are more generous, conforming as usual to the calibration of the roots. The narrow mesiodistal pulp cavity, however, will govern the initial entry of instruments. The labiolingual width of the cavity will be greater than that of the instrument; this must be kept in mind during debridement of soft tissue.

Since the two mandibular incisors are so nearly alike anatomically, the approach to endodontic treatment of the mandibular central incisor and the lateral incisor may be duplicated.

There is a possibility that the mandibular lateral incisor may have divided root canals more often than the central incisor (Fig. 9–14, 5, 6). Because such division occurs about midroot and is in a labiolingual direction, diagnosis of such a situation is most difficult.

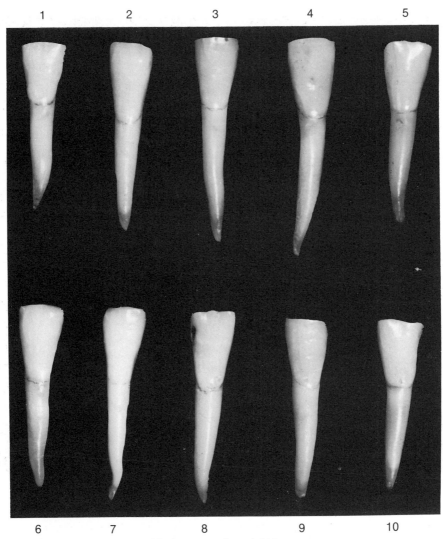

Figure 9–1 Mandibular central incisor—root form, labial aspect.

The mandibular central incisor crown has the smallest calibration mesiodistally of any tooth in the mouth. Therefore, its root is proportionately small in a mesiodistal direction. The widest calibration is at its union with the narrow crown at the cementoenamel junction. There it tapers rather evenly on both mesial and distal sides for two-thirds of its length, whereupon the taper is accelerated, ending in what appears to be a relatively sharp point. A look at the mesial or distal aspect of this mandibular incisor, however, will give a much different impression (Fig. 9–2). The root of this tooth is of good length, is usually well formed, and is often longer in a given case than the root of the *maxillary* central incisor.

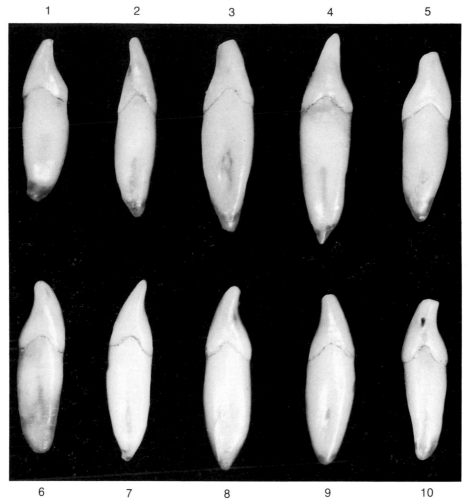

Figure 9-2   Mandibular central incisor—root form, mesial aspect.

Although the mandibular central incisor is quite small when compared to the other anterior teeth, from this aspect, the labiolingual measurement is quite substantial. The root at the cementoenamel junction is almost as wide as the crown in this view because mandibular anterior crowns have little or no enamel curvature labially or lingually at the cervical portion. This generous proportion labiolingually reinforces the small tooth in the directions in which masticatory forces must be withstood during functional activity. It also helps to avoid fracture from outside forces. The root form from mesial or distal aspects is as follows: labial and lingual sides will drop almost parallel to each other for over half the root length as they proceed apically. At approximately the dividing line between the middle third of the root and the apical third, the root tapers rapidly, coming to a blunt point at the apical end. Many of these teeth will have roots that have considerable breadth apically (6, 9) from this aspect. Quite possibly this type will have divided root canals, which must always be considered a possibility in endodontic diagnosis (Fig. 9-12, 3).

Figure 9–3 Mandibular central incisor, labial aspect and mesial aspect. The typical pulp cavity form is painted on the surfaces of the tooth as it might appear in cross section from the two aspects. Because the tooth is quite narrow in the mesiodistal calibration, the pulp chamber and pulp canal follow suit. The pulp chamber approximates the crown form in miniature; the pulp canal from the labial aspect is evenly slender like the tooth root. From the mesial aspect, the pulp cavity is large in a labiolingual direction. Here, also, the general outline of the pulp cavity copies the overall form of the whole tooth from this aspect (see Fig. 9–4, *A, D*).

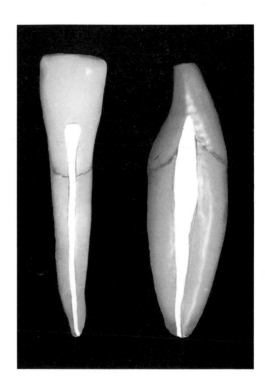

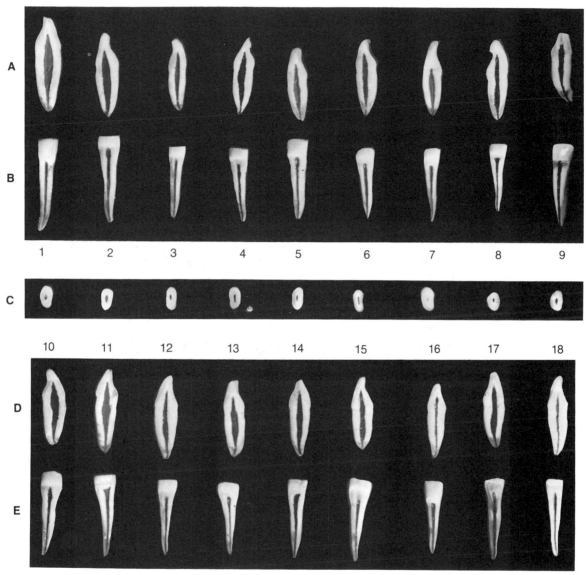

Figure 9–4   Mandibular central incisor (first incisor).

A, Labiolingual cross section, exposing the mesial or distal aspect of the pulp cavity. This aspect will not show on standard dental radiographs.

B, Mesiodistal cross section, exposing the labial or lingual aspect of the pulp cavity.

C, Cervical cross section. A transverse cut at the cementoenamel junction exposing the pulp chamber. These are the openings to root canals that will be seen in the floor of the pulp chamber.

D, Labiolingual cross section, exposing the mesial or distal aspect of the pulp cavity.

E, Mesiodistal cross section, exposing the labial or lingual aspect of the pulp cavity.

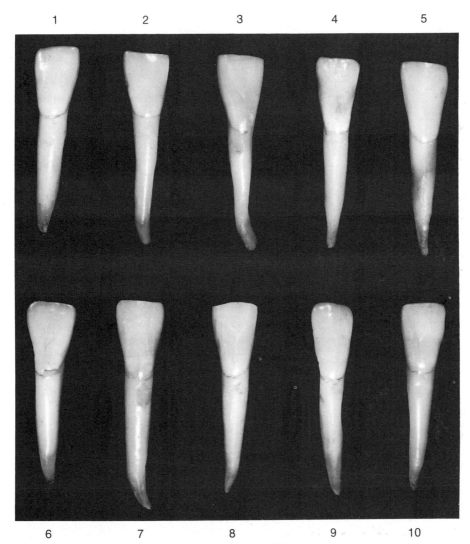

Figure 9–5 Mandibular lateral incisor—root form, labial aspect.

The description of the root form of the mandibular lateral incisor will be much like that of the mandibular central incisor. The two teeth are quite similar in size and shape because they function as a team. The root of the lateral incisor from this aspect may be a tiny fraction of a millimeter wider because its crown is approximately 0.5 mm wider mesiodistally. The general shape of the root of the lateral from the labial aspect is identical to that of the central. It may be a little longer and it may have a greater tendency for curvature at the apical end. It can curve mesially or distally. Radiographs taken with standard angulations will register a true picture of a given situation from this aspect.

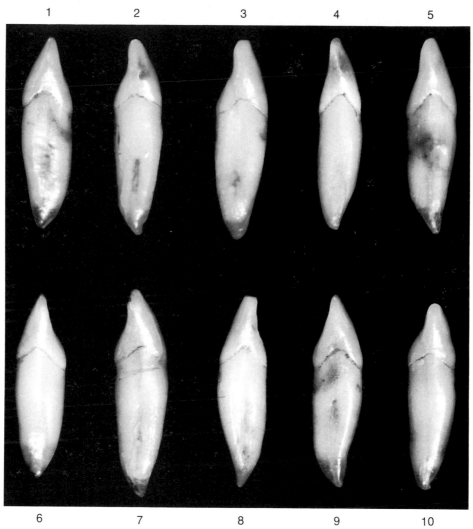

Figure 9–6 Mandibular lateral incisor—root form, mesial aspect.

Because the two teeth are so much alike, the description of the roots from the mesial aspect of the mandibular central incisor in the legend for Figure 9–2 is applicable to the mandibular lateral incisor roots as viewed from the mesial aspect. The lateral may show a little added root length, but the overall design from this aspect is identical.

Figure 9–7 Mandibular lateral incisor, mesial aspect and labial aspect.

The typical pulp cavity form is painted on the surfaces of the tooth as it might appear in cross section from the two aspects. In general, the pulp cavity form for the mandibular lateral incisor duplicates the mandibular central incisor form. If the labiolingual measurement of the lateral happens to be greater than usual labiolingually, which does happen sometimes, the pulp cavity would be wider in that dimension, which would indicate the housing of a little more soft tissue in vivo.

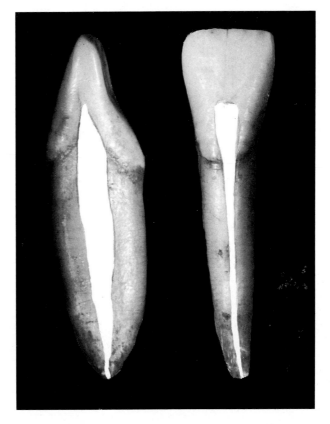

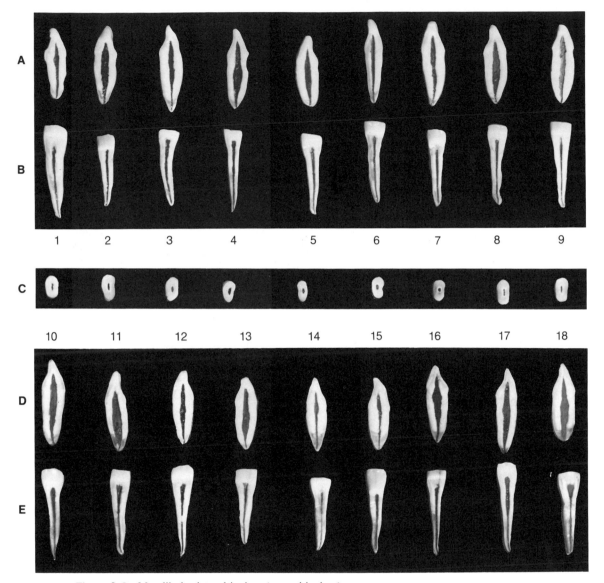

Figure 9–8   Mandibular lateral incisor (second incisor).
   A, Labiolingual cross section, exposing the mesial or distal aspect of the pulp cavity. This aspect will not show on the standard dental radiograph.
   B, Mesiodistal cross section, exposing the labial or lingual aspect of the pulp cavity.
   C, Cervical cross section. A transverse cut at the cementoenamel junction, exposing the pulp chamber. These are the openings to root canals that will be seen in the floor of the pulp chamber.
   D, Labiolingual cross section, exposing the mesial or distal aspect of the pulp cavity.
   E, Mesiodistal cross section, exposing the labial or lingual aspect of the pulp cavity.

Figure 9–9 A comparison of tooth form relations of the mandibular incisors.

1, Mandibular left central incisor, incisal aspect.

2, Mandibular left lateral incisor, incisal aspect.

The overall proportions of each tooth crown are shown in silhouette as they might be compared when sighting the teeth in line with their long axes. The enlargements are slightly in error in making the labiolingual and mesiodistal calibrations identical. The lateral should be a trifle larger in both measurements. However the alignment of crowns and roots is correct. The parallelism of the roots of the two teeth with the difference in the placement of the crowns on the roots is properly featured.

As pictured, the outlines of cervical areas are superimposed in white over the shaded crowns in a dimensional relationship. Pulp chamber openings are shaded also and are placed in proper relation to incisal surfaces. A broken line identifies the approximate location of the linguoincisal border of the incisal ridge in each of these teeth. It will be noted that the major portion of the pulp cavity will be located labial to this line. Therefore, an approach to the cavity from a lingual opening in the crown cannot be made in line with the pulp chamber and root canal (Figs. 9–10 and 9–11).

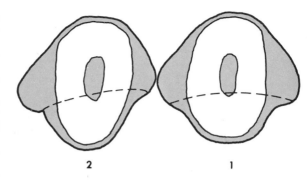

2   1

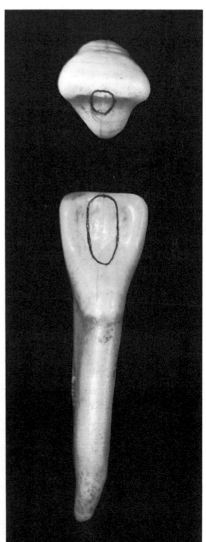

1

2

Figure 9–10 Mandibular central and lateral incisor.

1, Central incisor, incisal aspect, with marking outlining the centralized approach to the pulp cavity. If an indentation in the linguoincisal portion of the incisal ridge can be tolerated, as in this picture, it should be accomplished. Every effort should be made in the approach to the pulp chamber of either of the mandibular incisors to facilitate the placing of endodontic instruments in alignment with the entire pulp cavity (see Figs. 9–11 and 9–12).

2, Lateral incisor, with marking outlining the opening required for the proper approach to the pulp cavity. The area of outline is identical to the illustration above marking the mandibular central incisor. The broadside view of the lingual aspect as shown here will emphasize the total area to be included in the cut. If the specimen is posed so the view is exactly in line incisally with the long axis of the tooth, the marking will appear as in 1.

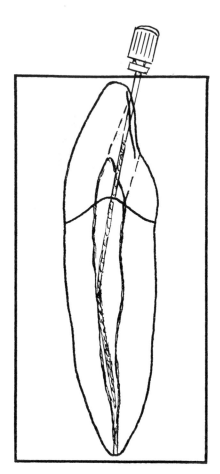

Figure 9–11 Mandibular incisor–approach to instrumentation.

A line drawing made by tracing the outline of an enlarged photograph of a mandibular incisor. The pulp cavity was drawn to represent one as it would appear in a labiolingual cross section (Fig. 9–4, *A*, 1). Broken lines extend from the pulp chamber to the linguoincisal surface of the crown and represent the opening suggested to allow the proper insertion of instruments for endodontic treatment. An instrument representing a root canal file has been inserted through the opening and projected until most of the pulp cavity appears to be penetrated. It will be noted that the shaft of the canal file is positioned tightly against the incisal ridge and the angle of entrance allows unobstructed travel into the tooth for only half the root length. Here it contacts the labial wall of the root canal and must bend considerably in order to continue apically. Understandably, this operation requires careful manipulation.

Figure 9–12 Mandibular central incisor.

1, *Mandibular central incisor* with a canal instrument placed in the canal through a lingual opening designed to save the incisal portion of the tooth. Note the angle of the instrument. 2, Photo of labiolingual section of this tooth. A straight probe is placed over a simulated lingual opening, showing the necessity for instrument flexibility in order to follow the pulp canal. 3, Photo of labiolingual cross section of another central incisor that had lost its incisal portion through abrasion. Note the "island" dividing the canal into labial and lingual portions. This situation is common but cannot be diagnosed from a radiograph taken with standard technique. A practical approach to the abraided type would be to enter the tooth through an opening in the incisal portion (note arrow).

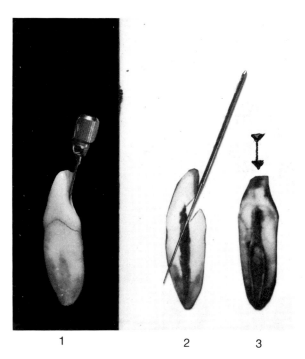

1   2   3

180

Figure 9–13 Mandibular central incisor—instrument approach to the pulp cavity.

Although these illustrations are of the mandibular central incisor, they could be used to illustrate the anatomy of the mandibular lateral incisor. As mentioned before, the root and pulp cavity anatomy of the two teeth for all practical purposes may be thought of as being identical.

This figure shows cut-outs of actual specimens of the mandibular central incisor. Simulated root canal instruments have been drawn to show the approach they would make as they entered root canals through suggested openings into the tooth crown as depicted in Figure 9–10. The specimen on the left is shown in a mesiodistal cross section as viewed from the labial aspect. The canal is narrow from this aspect, so the instrument appears to fill the canal, and it gives the impression of approaching the canal parallel to the root. The illustration on the right clearly shows the misapprehension in that belief. This specimen, showing the labiolingual cross section of a mandibular central incisor, has the simulated instrument entering the root canal at quite an angle. This is the mesial aspect of the specimen; the broad pulp cavity labiolingually is much wider than the instrument, and its approach does not include the pulp chamber roof, which seemed to be indicated by the picture on the left. The advisability of a dependency upon flexible root canal instruments, when treating difficult mandibular incisors, is unquestioned.

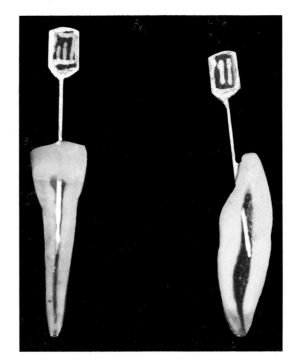

1   2   3   4   5   6

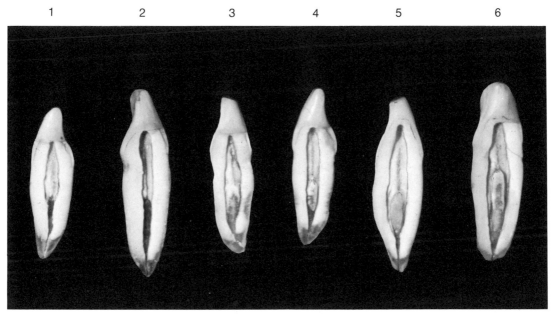

Figure 9–14   Mandibular central and lateral incisors, labiolingual cross sections.

Six well-formed specimens of mandibular central and lateral incisors intermixed. They are all good examples of pulp cavity anatomy which might be indicative of endodontic problems to be presented in the treatment of these teeth. 1 and 2 have single root canals extending the entire root length. The majority of mandibular incisors should be in this category. However, divided canals in the lower half of the root, labially and lingually, are common problems. Therefore, a special attempt was made to produce four examples (3, 4, 5, 6) which show the divided canal development. The obstruction that divides the canal looks like an "island" in a labiolingual cross section. Actually, in vivo with mesial and distal halves of the tooth joined, the obstruction is in the form of a "bar" joining the two halves. The pulp tissue divides and "jumps over" the bar. Discovering the presence of this type of root development in situ is most difficult. Standard procedure in dental radiography will not suffice.

It is possible that mandibular central incisors and especially lateral incisors that have greater than average labiolingual dimensions may be the types most likely to house divided root canals in the lower halves of the roots.

CHAPTER 10

Maxillary and Mandibular Canines

The maxillary and mandibular canines bear a close resemblance to each other, and their functions are closely related. Because of the shape of the crowns with their single, pointed cusps, their locations in the mouth, and the extra anchorage furnished by the long, strongly developed roots these teeth resemble those of the Carnivora; for this reason they are referred to as the canines.

Because of the labiolingual thickness of crown and root, and their anchorage in the alveolar process of the jaws, these teeth are perhaps the most stable in the mouth. The crown portions of the canines are shaped in a manner which promotes cleanliness. This self-cleansing quality, along with the efficient anchorage in the jaws, tends to preserve these teeth throughout life. When teeth are lost, the canines are usually the last to go. They are very valuable teeth, either as units of the natural dental arches or as possible assistants in stabilizing replacements of lost teeth in prosthetic procedures.

Both maxillary and mandibular canines have another quality which must not be overlooked: the position and forms of these teeth and their anchorage in the bone, along with the bone ridge over the labial portions of the roots, called the *canine eminence,* have a cosmetic value. They help to form a foundation that ensures normal facial expression at the corners of the mouth. Loss of all these teeth makes it extremely difficult, if not impossible, to make replacements that will restore the natural appearance of the face for any length of time. It would therefore be difficult to place a value on the canines, their importance being made manifest by their efficiency and function, stability, and help in maintaining natural facial expression.

Although the canines are more stable than other teeth in the mouth, still there are times when they require endodontic treatment. Endodontic treatment is accomplished more easily in the canines than in any other teeth. The pulp cavities are more generous

183

in size because of the large root calibrations; this is especially true of the maxillary canines.

Ease of access is usually characteristic of the mandibular canine also, but at times this tooth can present problems. On many occasions the mandibular canine will have a bifurcated root and consequently a divided root canal. This situation cannot always be anticipated because the standard radiograph technique may not register the situation on the dental film (Figs. 10–19 and 10–20).

MAXILLARY CANINE

CALCIFICATION OF THE MAXILLARY CANINE

First evidence of calcification	4 to 5 months
Enamel completed	6 to 7 years
Eruption	11 to 12 years
Root completed	13 to 15 years

CROSS-SECTIONAL ANATOMY: DESIGN OF PULP CAVITIES (Fig. 10–4, *A, B, C, D, E*)

Labiolingual Cross Section (Fig. 10–4, *A, D*)

The labiolingual measurement of the maxillary canine root registers the largest root calibration in width of any tooth in the mouth. Therefore, the pulp cavity will be very generous in size labiolingually (Fig. 10–3). Ordinarily, the extra width to accommodate a bulk of pulp tissue will be shown in most of these canines in the half of the root closest to the crown because the canal at that point is continuous with the pulp chamber of the crown. The apical half of the pulp canal should narrow to average width toward the apical end of the root. Nevertheless, some variations will be found in this typical form of pulp cavity. Those that do not conform will usually show a generous labiolingual measurement for the entire root length (Fig. 10–4, *A*, 3, 7, 9; *D*, 10).

The problems of endodontic treatment can be multiplied if the operator fails to remember the details in pulp cavity anatomy displayed by labiolingual cross sections of canines. Endodontic manipulation must take into consideration the need for removal of a bulk of soft tissue in the maxillary canine; after that removal, there will be problems associated with the preparation and filling of the wide, oddly shaped root canal. It must be emphasized again that the standard technique in radiography will not give a true picture of the labiolingual aspect of anterior teeth. A diagnosis of the local condition must be made clinically (Figs. 10–8 and 10–9).

Mesiodistal Cross Section (Fig. 10–4, *B, E*)

The pulp cavity seems much narrower when viewing this section. Other than its length, it compares favorably with the other maxillary anterior teeth in shape. It must be remembered that the maxillary canine possesses the longest root in the dentition.

Since the mesiodistal measurement of the root is less than the labiolingual measurement, the pulp canal in this section will be narrower also. If constriction of the canal is discovered in one of these teeth, it is very likely to be in a mesiodistal direction (Fig. 10–4, *B*, 3; *E*, 13). The shape of the root canal is elliptical rather than round, with the long calibration labiolingually (Fig. 10–9, *A*, *B*).

Cervical Cross Section (Fig. 10–4, *C*)

The pulp cavity quite typically is centered in the root of the maxillary canine. Generally speaking, the outline of the periphery of the cavity will duplicate the root form in miniature. The root of the maxillary canine is wider labially than it is lingually; therefore, the greater width labially is reflected in the calibration of the width of the root canal labially. Also, since the root is narrower mesiodistally than labiolingually, the pulp chamber and root canal adapt to this form. As mentioned before, constriction of the canal would most likely be in a mesiodistal direction (Fig. 10–4, *C*, 1, 3).

MANDIBULAR CANINE

CALCIFICATION OF THE MANDIBULAR CANINE

First evidence of calcification	4 to 5 years
Enamel completed	6 to 7 years
Eruption	9 to 10 years
Root completed	12 to 14 years

CROSS-SECTIONAL ANATOMY: DESIGN OF PULP CAVITIES (Fig. 10–14, *A, B, C, D, E*)

Labiolingual Cross Section (Fig. 10–14, *A, D*)

The pulp cavity in this cross section of the mandibular canine compares favorably in size and shape with that of the maxillary canine. This might be expected, since the dimensions of the two teeth labiolingually are similar, although not identical. The maxillary canine is usually about 0.5 mm wider in that calibration. The pulp chamber is pointed incisally and sometimes appears with a rounded roof later in life; the pulp canal is quite wide labiolingually in the main portion of the root, narrowing at about the halfway point in the root heading toward the apex (Fig. 10–14, *A*, 1, 5, 6). Other canines will show the constriction of the canal in the apical third only (Fig. 10–14, *A*, 3, 7; *D*, 10, 14). In all broad-rooted teeth (including the canines), one may find an "island" in the center of the broadest portion. This form creates a "double" canal on the sides of the obstruction until the canal becomes single again as it approaches the apex of the root (Fig. 10–14, *A*, 4). Some canines are quite large and long, whereas others are smaller than average. Mandibular canines tend to be shorter than maxillary canines. Very short canines may be present only in individuals with slender mandibles. Although it is not frequently anticipated, the mandibular canine can be longer than the maxillary canine. If that should be true, the pulp cavity would vary accordingly (Fig. 10–14, *B*, 9).

There is one outstanding anatomical variation in the mandibular canine: it is not uncommon to find that this tooth has two roots, or at least a fused root with two canals in the root portion, one labial and one lingual. The pulp cavity in a tooth of this kind would vary accordingly if a labiolingual cross section were to be examined (see Fig. 10–20, *C*). The anomalies do not always show on radiographs; *consequently, great care must be observed in searching for the possibility of two root canals when the mandibular canine is under treatment.*

Mesiodistal Cross Section (Fig. 10–14, *B*, *E*)

Generally speaking, when viewing the mesiodistal cross section of the mandibular canines, it is immediately apparent from this aspect that this tooth is similar to the maxillary canine. The cross section will be a little narrower mesiodistally, but the root will appear quite long and may show some curvature at the apical portion. The curvature can be directed either mesially or distally. Oddly enough, the curvature will be in a mesial direction most often (Fig. 10–11, 1, 2, 3, 4).

The root canal from this aspect appears narrow with rather straight sides for the full length of the root until it becomes more constricted as it approaches its apex.

Cervical Cross Section (Fig. 10–14, *C*)

The cervical cross section of the mandibular canine shows some variations in size and shape of the root when comparing several specimens. The root canal is centered as usual and takes on the general shape, much diminished of course, of the root outline from this aspect. Some roots will be smoothly oblong, with the greatest measurement labiolingually; others will show proportions closer to the maxillary canine, with calibration of the lingual portion of the root appearing less than that of the labial portion (Fig. 10–14, *C*, 2, 3, 9). Usually the pulp cavity of the mandibular canine will be readily accessible in endodontic treatment. Exceptions may always be found, of course (Fig. 10–14, *C*, 5; *E*, 14).

SUMMARY — MAXILLARY AND MANDIBULAR CANINES

Anatomically, the maxillary and the mandibular canines have much in common because they have similar functions. Their smooth forms and strong, well-developed roots ensure their usefulness and guarantee their long life.

When teeth are lost, the canines are usually the last to go. They are very valuable as stabilizing units when the dental arches are complete and also as stabilizers for prosthetic restorations when other teeth have been lost.

Their cosmetic value must not be discounted; along with the prominence of canine eminences labial to the roots, these teeth help to form the bony foundation which ensures normal facial expression at the corners of the mouth.

It would be difficult to place a value on the canines. Although more stable than other teeth in the arches, endodontic treatment will be needed at times. Because the pulp cavities are generous in size as a result of large root calibrations, endodontic manipulation is usually uneventful. The mandibular canine may present a problem; it may have a bifurcated root or divided root canals that might not be revealed in a standard dental radiograph (Fig. 10–20, *B, C*).

1   2   3   4   5

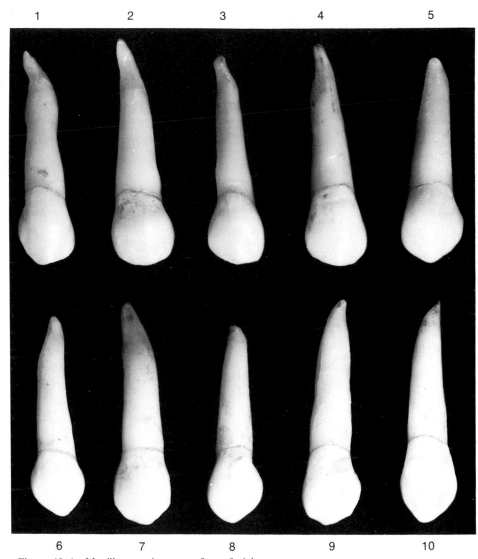

6   7   8   9   10

Figure 10-1 Maxillary canine—root form, facial aspect.

As a rule, the maxillary canine root is the longest and the strongest to be found in the permanent dentition. The mesiodistal measurement of the root even near the base of the crown is likely to be a millimeter less than that of the maxillary central incisor but quite sturdy nevertheless. From the facial aspect, the root tapers gradually, coming to a blunt point at the apical end. The root can be relatively straight from this aspect, or it may bend slightly to the distal at the apical third. Warning : the clinician may be thrown off guard by the standard dental radiograph that would corroborate the statement on root curvature. Studies of the *mesial* aspects of canine roots, including those sectioned faciolingually, will show a sharper curvature of the same teeth in a *facial* direction in many instances (Figs. 10-2, 1 and 10-4, *A*, 3, 7). The anchorage afforded by the husky root of the maxillary canine and the smooth hygienic form of the tooth crown assures the permanency of this most valuable dental unit.

1   2   3   4   5

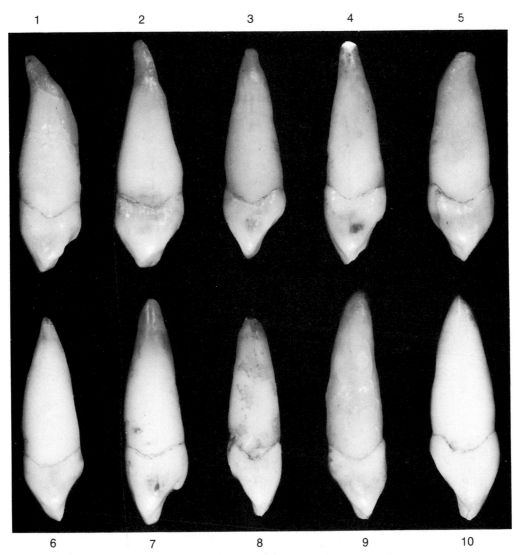

6   7   8   9   10

Figure 10-2 Maxillary canine — root form, mesial aspect.

Generally speaking, from this aspect the canine root is conical with a tapered or bluntly pointed apex. The labial outline of the root usually will present a straighter line than that marking the lingual border. In other words, the labial outline of the root may be almost perpendicular, with most of the root taper appearing on the lingual side. The shape of a pulp cavity tends to follow in miniature the shape of crown and root. There is one other anatomical detail that is characteristic of the maxillary canine and that differs from other maxillary anterior teeth: the tooth crown is set on the root in a different relationship to root axis. From the mesial or distal aspect, a line which would bisect the cusp tip will usually be labial to a line bisecting the root. Lines bisecting the roots of *maxillary incisors* would bisect the incisal ridges. With the arrrangement characteristic of the canine, opening the crown lingually to gain access for endodontic instrumentation is facilitated. Instruments may be introduced more nearly in line with the root canal without cutting into the cusp ridges of the canine (Figs. 10–8, 2 and 10–10, *B*).

From the mesial aspect, the canine roots are very broad with a developmental indentation of fluting extending for most of the root length. This form increases the anchorage efficiency by preventing rotation in alveolar bone. The specimens in this figure were chosen as examples of those approaching the ideal in size and form. It must be kept in mind that there can be size differentials, particularly in canines in different individuals (Fig. 10–6). This would be significant in contemplating possible root length in treatment. Sometimes the maxillary canine will have a root much longer than the crown size would indicate (Fig. 10–4, *B*, 1; *D*, 10).

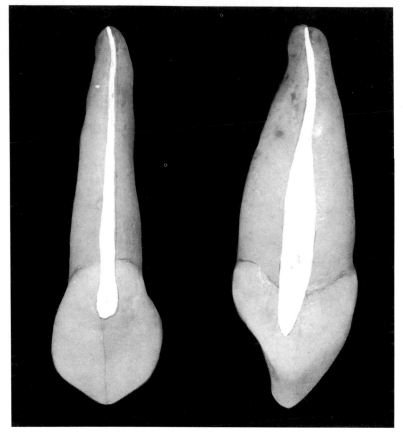

Figure 10–3 Maxillary canine, facial* aspect and mesial aspect.

The typical pulp cavity form is painted on the surfaces of the tooth as it might appear in cross section from the two aspects.

From the *facial* aspect, the pulp chamber and pulp canal follow the regular and rather narrow tooth form, the widest point located in the crown and cervical third of the root. From that area, the taper is gradual, the canal, as usual, becoming quite small, as the apical end of the root is approached.

From the *mesial* aspect, the pulp cavity can be rather wide in a faciolingual direction for most of its length. The pointed pulp chamber portion is continuous with the broad canal in the cervical portion, narrowing in the apical third on the way to the apical foramen. Seemingly, there are three pulp cavity forms as viewed from the mesial aspect (Fig. 10–4):

1, The wide portion is confined to the cervical third portions of crown and root (Fig. 10–4, *A*, 1, 4, 8).

2, The wide portion of the pulp cavity will extend from the crown to the middle third of the root (Fig. 10–4, *A*, 5, 6; *D*, 10).

3. The wide portion will make up most of the root length with a tendency to include a generous approach to the root end (Fig. 10–4, *A*, 3, 7, 9).

Usually the process of gaining access to and penetrating the pulp cavity of the maxillary canine will be uneventful. Except in patients who are quite old with overcalcified teeth, the manipulation of root canal instruments will be unobstructed (Fig. 10–8).

---

*Because the canines can qualify anatomically as teeth with both anterior and posterior functions, it was decided to use the term facial here to serve as a combination of the terms labial and buccal.

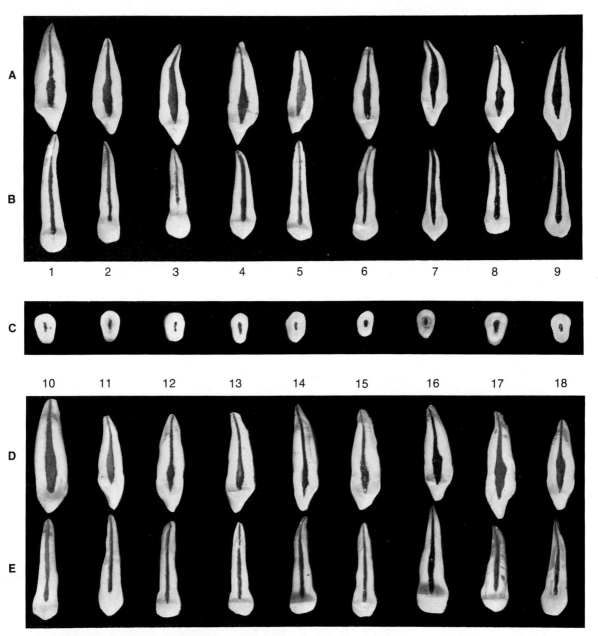

Figure 10–4 Maxillary canine.

A, Labiolingual cross section, exposing the mesial or distal aspect of the pulp cavity. This aspect does not show in dental radiographs taken in the usual manner.

B, Mesiodistal cross section, exposing the labial or lingual aspect of the pulp cavity.

C, Cervical cross section. A transverse cut at the cementoenamel junction exposing the pulp chamber. These are the openings to root canals that will be seen in the floor of the pulp chamber.

D, Labiolingual cross section, exposing the mesial or distal aspect of the pulp cavity.

E, Mesiodistal cross section, exposing the labial or lingual aspect of the pulp cavity.

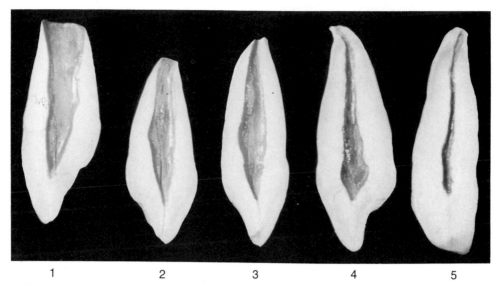

Figure 10–5 Labiolingual sections showing various stages of development of the maxillary canine. 1, Crown complete, root partially completed with large pulp cavity, wide open at the apical end. 2, Tooth almost complete except for lack of constriction of apical foramen. 3, Canine of young individual with large pulp cavity and complete root tip with generous foramen. 4, Typical average canine in adult stage with constricted apical foramen. 5, Canine of an old individual with constricted pulp chamber and canal; it will be noted that this specimen has lost its original crown form through wear and erosion.

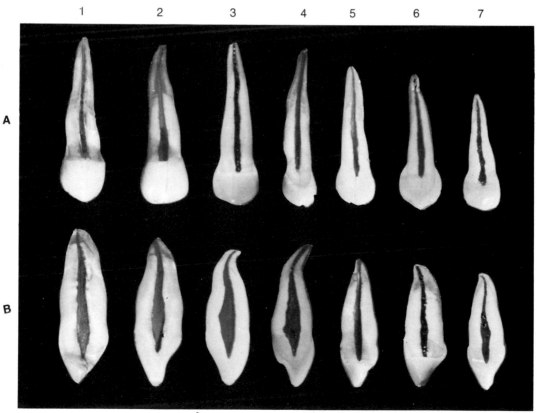

Figure 10–6 *See opposite page for legend.*

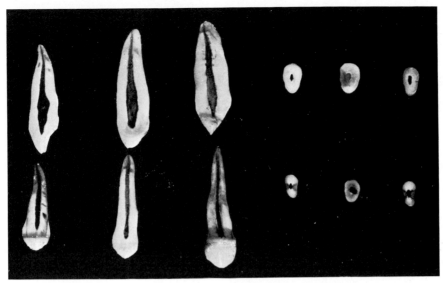

Figure 10–7 Variations in the size and shape of cross sections of canines.
Top row, labiolingual sections of maxillary canines with cervical sections to the right. The pulp cavities shown demonstrate the three types from this aspect mentioned in Figure 10–3, 1, 2, 3.
Bottom row, mesiodistal sections of canines of similar size, flanked by midroot sections.

Figure 10–6 Maxillary canine, mesiodistal cross sections and faciolingual cross sections. These 14 well-formed typical cross sections of the maxillary canine were chosen to add perspective to the present study. The two rows were graded in size to show the probabilities that might be involved in the study of size differentials.

A, Mesiodistal cross sections. Note the size gradations including the variance in root length; yet the root canals are of rather even width, straight with an even taper. Two specimens are of special interest: 7 has a root that is quite short and yet the crown portion is as large as or larger than specimen 4, which has a root attached to the small crown that is as long as any of the canines in the row, including those with large crowns and roots in good proportion.

B, Faciolingual cross sections. These specimens give a clear picture of the pulp cavity anatomy which could be encountered during endodontic procedure. None of the cavities from this aspect show any obstruction, and the first four are demonstrating wide cavity formations in a faciolingual direction. Note the tendency of all of them to lean facially as the apical region is approached; two are curved markedly.

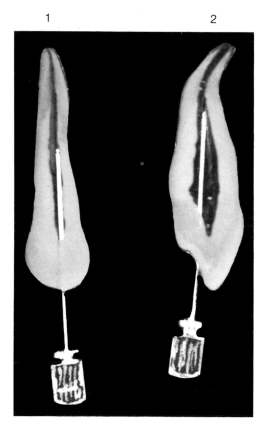

1   2

Figure 10–8 Maxillary canine, cross sections indicating instrument approach. Two cross sections of the maxillary canine with simulated root canal instruments drawn to show the angles of insertion as they enter the canal with two aspects of the tooth involved.

1, Mesiodistal cross section. From this aspect the canal appears quite straight. The instrument would be placed in the lingual opening to the pulp chamber, keeping the shaft of the instrument in line with the tip of the canine cusp. The mesial and distal walls would not interfere with the further penetration of the instrument. The facial or lingual walls might, however.

2, Faciolingual cross section. The instrumentation presents different problems from this aspect. First, the instrument is involved with a space more extensive than that found in the mesiodistal cross section. Although it approaches the lingual wall of the root canal, it is far away from the facial wall. When the pulp cavity is filled with pulp tissue, the removal of it will not be gained by an operator unfamiliar with this situation. The technique of removal will have to be adapted to the problem. A further look at the drawing of the instrument as it travels root-wise indicates a stoppage at some point where the pulp cavity wall is curved as it approaches its terminal. Usually, in cases similar to this, the collision will occur near the apical third of the root. This would suggest the use of flexible instruments until penetration reaches the apical end of the cavity. If very much curvature is involved, as in this illustration, care must be used in order to avoid blockage or a "false canal" which could spell failure for the operator.

As mentioned earlier, a maxillary canine could present a straight root from the facial aspect, as shown in 1 of this figure; and then if it were possible to view the root from the mesial in a radiograph, it could show curvature facially at the apical third, just as extreme as in specimen 2 (Fig. 10–6, *B*, 2, 3, 4).

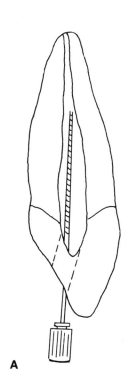

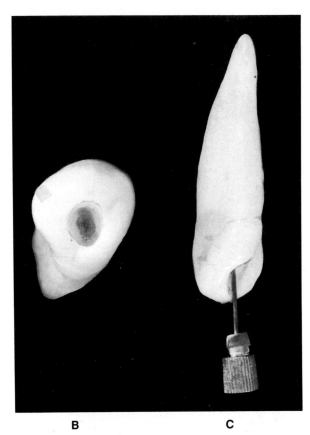

Figure 10–9 Maxillary canine, instrument approach in endodontic manipulation.

A, A drawing of a maxillary canine that demonstrates the relationship of root canal instrument to pulp cavity walls. When access is gained through the lingual surface of the tooth, it is possible to create an opening into the pulp chamber that is nearly in line with the center of the root (Fig. 10–10). A straight instrument will possibly penetrate two-thirds of the root canal before it is challenged by a cavity wall. The maxillary canine differs from other single-rooted maxillary teeth in its alignment of pulp cavity with its incisal portion (Fig. 10–10, *B*).

B, Linguo-occlusal view of a maxillary canine specimen with a properly placed opening into the pulp chamber. The opening into the pulp cavity seems to be perfectly centered, but the view in perspective of the root portion of the specimen shows the tooth to be posed so that the cusp and cusp ridges are not centered with the long axis.

C, A root canal file is placed in a natural specimen of a maxillary canine, copying the approach toward manipulation shown by the drawing in *A*. The instrument is directly against the incisal margin of the lingual opening.

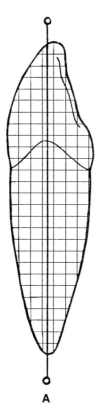

A

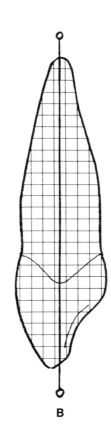

B

Figure 10–10 Maxillary and mandibular canines—a comparison.

These two paste-ups of tooth outlines are intended to show the relationship of the tooth crowns to the root bases and to the long axes of the maxillary and the mandibular canines. In this relationship, the two teeth are not formed exactly alike, which changes the plan of approach somewhat when initial entry is made linguoincisally into the pulp chamber for endodontic treatment.

A, The mandibular canine, mesial aspect. A line is drawn, bisecting the root, and is continued through the crown, ending beyond the tip of the cusp. All mandibular anterior teeth, including the canine, will show a tendency, as in this case, for the cusp tip and incisal ridges to be *lingual* to a line bisecting the root from the mesial or distal aspect. In these teeth, the approach to the pulp cavity with the opening lingual to the cusp tip will increase the difficulty of inserting root canal instruments (Figs. 10–17 and 10–18).

B, The maxillary canine, mesial aspect. Here, as in *A*, a line is drawn bisecting the root and continued beyond the cusp tip of the crown. The maxillary canine differs from the mandibular by having its cusp tip *labial* to the bisecting line. This formation facilitates instrument manipulation to some extent. The linguoincisal opening can be made nearer to the pulp canal alignment without encroaching upon the cusp. The introduction of instruments will be more nearly in line with the axis (Fig. 10–9, *A*).

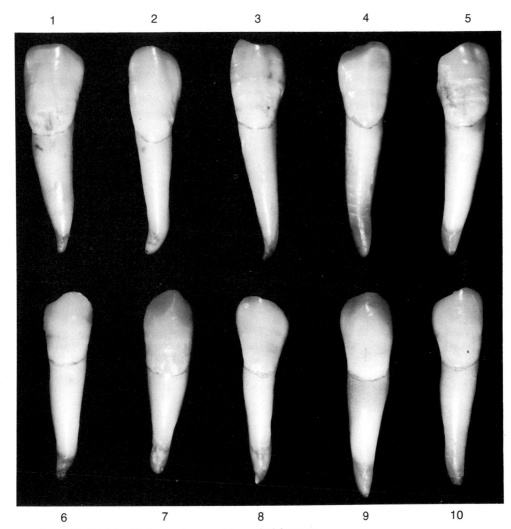

Figure 10–11 Mandibular canine—root form, facial aspect.

The mandibular canine root, like the maxillary, is large and well formed, affording excellent anchorage at the lower corner of the mouth. The root is usually slightly shorter than that of the maxillary canine in the same mouth, but as with any anatomical comparisons, this statement cannot be accepted as a fixed rule. Averages in tooth measurements will favor this statement; however, both canines will have approximately the same overall length, with the *crown* of the *mandibular canine* a millimeter or so longer than the maxillary, and the *root* of the *maxillary canine* a millimeter or so longer than that of the mandibular (Fig. 10–10). Usually, the mesiodistal measurement of crown and root of the mandibular canine is a little less than that of the maxillary tooth and, with a tendency to be somewhat shorter, the mandibular canine root with its rapid taper toward the apex gives the impression of being smaller than it is at times. The generous length of the crown portion of the tooth adds to the illusion. From the labial aspect the roots seem quite pointed at their apical ends, with sudden curvature apically in a *mesial* direction in the majority of cases.

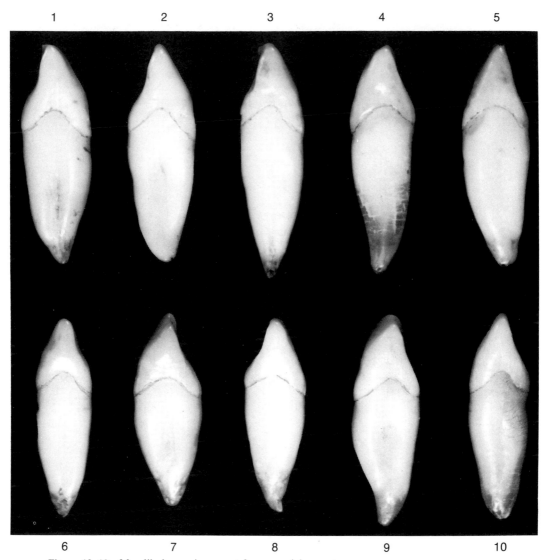

Figure 10–12   Mandibular canine — root form, mesial aspect.
The mesial aspect of the mandibular canine is quite similar to that of the maxillary canine with the possible exception of a more pointed root tip. The faciolingual measurements of the roots of both teeth are approximate, making the roots quite thick and sturdy. This design resists the displacement of the canine, giving it security even when unusual stresses are encountered. The canines are designed not only to protect themselves but to act as guards and protectors of neighboring teeth, both mesially and distally. The teeth in this figure were chosen as average representatives. Therefore, another illustration must be consulted in order to study variations that are not rare in mandibular canine roots, such as fused roots and bifurcated roots that contain branching pulp cavities (Figs. 10–19 and 10–20).

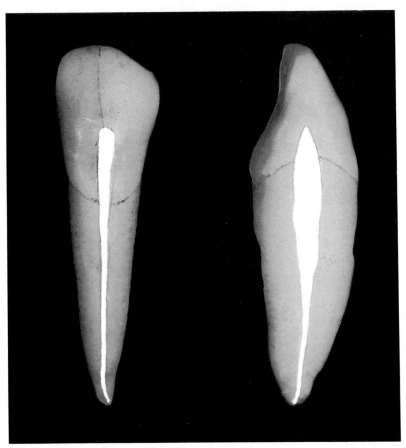

Figure 10–13   Mandibular canine, facial* aspect, and mesial aspect.

The typical pulp cavity form is painted on the surfaces of the tooth as it might appear in cross section from the two aspects.

From the facial aspect, the pulp chamber and pulp canal follow the regular and rather narrow tooth form, the wider portion appearing in the crown and in the cervical third of the root. From the cervical third of the root, the taper of the canal is gradual, becoming quite narrow as the apical end of the root is approached.

From the mesial aspect, the pulp cavity that includes the pulp chamber in the crown portion can be quite wide in a faciolingual direction until midroot is reached. Usually it narrows considerably in this area, becoming more constricted as it continues its journey, terminating as a small apical foramen at the root end. This is a composite picture of what is to be expected in the average case. Other illustrations in this chapter will picture other probabilities (Fig. 10–14, *A, D*).

---

*Because the canines can qualify anatomically as teeth with both anterior and posterior functions, it was decided to use the term facial here to serve as a combination of the terms labial and buccal.

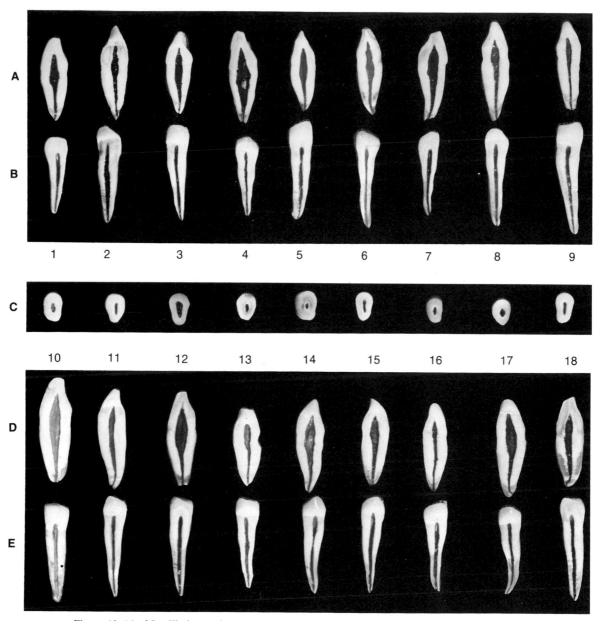

Figure 10–14   Mandibular canine.

A, Labiolingual cross section, exposing the mesial or distal aspect of the pulp cavity. This aspect will not show on dental radiographs taken in the usual manner.

B, Mesiodistal cross section, exposing the labial or lingual aspect of the pulp cavity.

C, Cervical cross section. A transverse cut at the cementoenamel junction, exposing the pulp chamber. These are the openings to root canals that will be seen in the floor of the pulp chamber.

D, Labiolingual cross section, exposing the mesial or distal aspect of the pulp cavity.

E, Mesiodistal cross section, exposing the labial or lingual aspect of the pulp cavity.

A   **B**

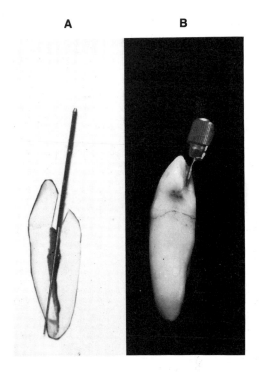

Figure 10–15 Mandibular canine — instrument approach to the pulp cavity.

A, Labiolingual cross section of a mandibular canine with a small portion cut away lingually, simulating a cut to gain access to the pulp cavity. A straight smooth broach was placed over the photo, visualizing the limitation of entry into the root canal and how it was impeded by the labial cavity wall. This illustration emphasizes the need for care in the manipulation of *flexible* instruments in this situation.

B, A natural tooth specimen of a mandibular canine posed to parallel the specimen in *A.* Lingual access to the pulp cavity has been attained, and a root canal file has been inserted into the tooth until stopped by the labial wall of the root canal. This is further proof of the need for care and a working knowledge of the cross-sectional anatomy when treating the mandibular canine.

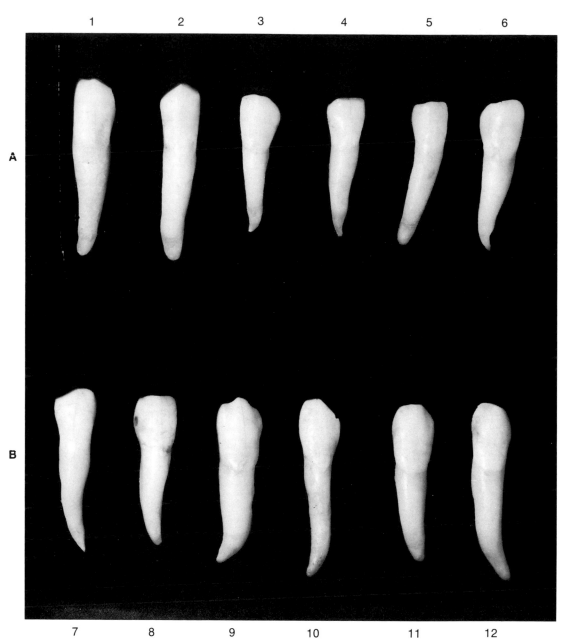

Figure 10–16 Mandibular canine – 12 excellent specimens considered to be normal.

A, The six specimens in the upper row differ in size and in some minor details, but they have one thing in common – the roots are relatively straight from the root base to root tip.

B, The six specimens in the lower row have a common trait – each root shows definite curvature apically; most of them curve mesially (7, 8, 9, 10); two curve distally (11, 12). Many think this is the proportionate curvature to be expected in the mandibular canine roots.

Figure 10–17 Mandibular canine, cross sections, indicating instrument approach.

Two cross sections of the mandibular canine with simulated root canal instruments drawn to show the angles of insertion from two aspects as they enter the pulp cavity through a linguoincisal opening.

1, Mesiodistal cross section. From this aspect the cavity appears straight and quite slender. If the pointed cusp is present (this one was worn away), the instrument would be inserted in line with the point of the cusp. The mesial and distal walls would not interfere with further penetration, but facial or lingual walls might, as will be indicated by the faciolingual cross section on the right. The specimen under discussion displays a comparatively straight root. However, many mandibular canines will have a root with its canal showing more curvature mesially at the apical third (Fig. 10–16).

2, Faciolingual cross section. This specimen compares favorably in being average anatomically. The pulp cavity form can be considered average for the mandibular canine from this aspect. The incisal ridge is lingual of root center. The latter relationship is usual, but not invariable (see Fig. 10–10). When a root canal instrument is inserted into the linguoincisal opening, the operator usually inserts it in line with the labial face of the tooth. If this is to be the case, the faciolingual cross section under discussion will show why progress of the instrument will be limited. Tipping the instrument labially in a canal as wide as this one will afford further penetration to a limited degree before striking the labial wall of the cavity a little farther down (Fig. 10–18).

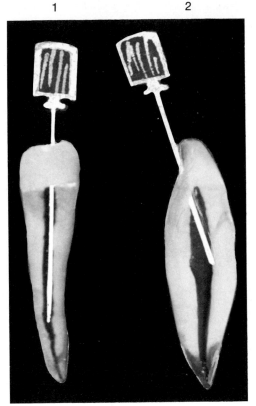

1 2

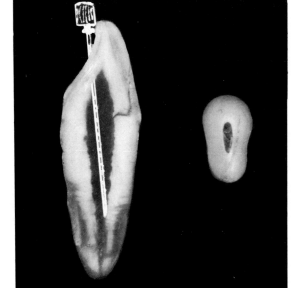

Figure 10–18 Mandibular canine, faciolingual cross section and cervical root section.

The faciolingual cross section shown here is of a choice specimen of mandibular canine that displays a broad, well-formed pulp cavity conforming to what might be called the ideal development. A tooth like this would be of considerable assistance to the endodontist who is contemplating its treatment. The specimen showed signs of erosion and incisal wear, so the open pulp cavity was viewed with some surprise. The drawing of a simulated canal in Figure 10–13 will demonstrate the relative sizes when the two are compared.

The cervical cross section to the right shows a nearly perfect specimen of a root cross section of a mandibular canine cut at the cementoenamel junction facially and lingually. The root is wider facially than lingually, with some developmental constriction mesially and distally, which adds to the magnificent retention in the alveolus enjoyed by a well-formed mandibular canine. The open root canal is centered and tends to copy the root form in miniature.

203

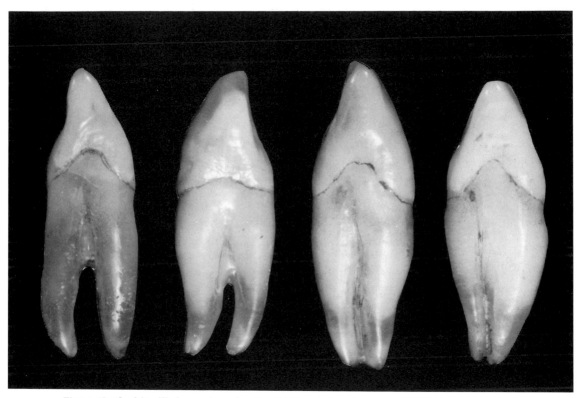

Figure 10–19   Mandibular canine—fused and bifurcated roots.

Because the oddity occurs quite often and because many endodontic treatment failures have been due to the lack of discovery of this anomaly in the diagnosis of given cases, this figure is provided for special emphasis. These four outstanding specimens show graphically the maldevelopment of the mandibular canine which can and does take place. The first two shown are bifurcated completely; the final two have two roots joined together. The standard dental radiograph will not register this anomaly clearly enough to be distinguishable. However, if the clinician is aware of probabilities, the true state of affairs can be ascertained by "following up" on suspicious leads in diagnosis.

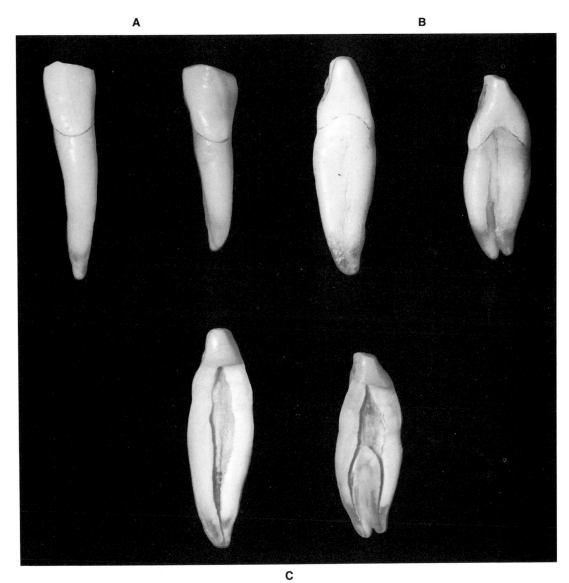

Figure 10–20 Mandibular canine, normal and abnormal—comparing two outstanding specimens.

A, Two mandibular canine specimens, labial aspect. The specimen on the left is a nearly perfect representative, with crown and root properly proportioned. The specimen on the right appears to be well formed with a possible exception: the root seems a little short compared to crown length.

B, The mesial aspect of the two specimens shown in *A* displays them in "true colors." The left tooth is normal in every way, whereas the one on the right has a normal crown form, but its root, although strong, is a little short and definitely bifurcated.

C, Both teeth shown in *A* and *B* have been dissected in a labiolingual direction. The resulting cross sections display the respective pulp cavities perfectly. Both are representative of what the endodontist is likely to find in the two types.

The two teeth as shown in *A,* before dissection, are posed to show the profile registration to be expected on a standard dental radiograph. Although on the one, the bifurcation shows a tiny bit at the root end, it would be very easy to overlook that detail in the radiographic diagnosis.

Index

Note: Page numbers in *italics* refer to illustrations.

207